MICHAEL VAN STRATEN

Guarana

The Energy Seeds and Herbs of the Amazon Rainforest

Index compiled by
Jenny Knight

SAFFRON WALDEN
THE C. W. DANIEL COMPANY LIMITED

First published in Great Britain in 1994
by The C. W. Daniel Company Limited
1 Church Path, Saffron Walden
Essex, CB10 1JP, England

© Michael van Straten

ISBN 0 85207 263 5

This book is printed on part-recycled paper

Produced in association with
Book Production Consultants, Plc
Typeset in Adobe Garamond
by KeyStar, St Ives, Cambridgeshire
and printed by St Edmundsbury Press,
Bury St Edmunds, Suffolk

Guarana

Contents

Dedication

For Bira my guide in the rainforest, his mother – one of the best cooks I've ever met – for the wonderful friendly people on the River Amazon, for the villagers in the forest and their hospitality, for Amazonino Mendes, now mayor of Manaus, and most of all for Sally, whom I should have been with when I went to the rainforest.

This book is also dedicated to Graeme, Denise and Ben. They didn't make the great mistake but started by doing a little. They are now doing more than most to ensure the survival of the Brazilian rainforest, the people who live there, the cornucopia of potential benefits for mankind that flourish under its canopy and the medicine men who have knowledge to share.

'Nobody makes a greater mistake than he who did nothing because he could only do a little.'

Edmund Burke, Statesman and orator

'Each time a medicine man dies, it's as if a library has burned down.'

Mark Plotkin, World Wide Fund for Nature

Foreword

'The Lord hath created medicines out of the earth; and he that is wise will not abhor them'.

Ecclesiasticus, 38:4

From pre-history to modern days mankind has made use of plant medicines which grow 'out of the earth'. The history of medicine is filled with the names of great pioneers who used these plants in their efforts to alleviate suffering. The Roman physician Dioscorides remained the authority on medicinal plants for 1,500 years. Culpeper, whose *Herbal* was published in 1649, made simple remedies available to physicians and patients alike. The Reverend Edward Stone in 1758 discovered the pain-killing properties of the bark of the white willow tree; and Felix Hoffman developed aspirin from *Spirea*, the meadowsweet widely used by herbalists. Jesse Boot, who left school at the age of 13 to help in his mother's herbal shop in Nottingham, had more than a thousand shops when he died in 1931. Russell Marker and his colleagues Karl Djerassi and George Rosenkrantz succeeded in creating 'The Pill' from a strain of wild yam which grows in Mexico.

Some botanists believe that there are up to thirty thousand plant species in the Brazilian rainforest, and statistically around 10% of these, a staggering three thousand plants, are likely to have medicinal benefits. I have attempted here to tell you something of the few plants which we so far know have valuable properties. I hope that this tantalising glimpse of the hidden magic in the rainforest will stimulate further research and will add more fuel to the flames of the growing number of voices raised in protest against the destruction of this unique, valuable and environmentally vital treasure trove of nature's bounty.

Introduction

Healing herbs
from the rainforest

We have a lot to learn about the medicinal value of plants from the
Indians in Brazil.

If we continue to destroy the rainforest, we will be depriving
mankind of potential medical benefits which are beyond our
wildest dreams. Cures for cancer, AIDS, lupus, leukaemia
and who knows what else, could be going up in smoke as
thousands of plants are being wiped off the face of the
Earth.

These were the opening words from ethnobotanist Dr Walter
Accorsi, professor of botany at São Paulo University, when we met
in Brazil. He is the founder of the Brazilian Ethnobotanical Society
and director of the Medicinal Plant Research Laboratory at the university, and a passionate worker for the protection of the rainforest
flora.

Is it too late? Thanks to the efforts of a handful of far-sighted
people, hopefully not. One of these is a young Englishman,
Graeme Lewis, who went to Brazil for a holiday, lived for two years
on a remote island, and fell under the spell of the Amazon, its people, and its plants. He determined to try to help, so he began
importing some of the Indian herbal medicines to England. I went
with him to the rainforest to find out more about one of the most
effective of the traditional remedies, Guarana.

Our journey took us on a sixteen-hour flight to the town of Manaus, in the Amazon basin, then by boat down the river to the small village of Maués – thirty hours of gentle meandering on the Amazon itself – and finally through a maze of smaller tributaries. No matter what you have read, heard or seen about the Amazon and the rainforest, nothing prepares you for the first sights, sounds and smells. The majesty of a waterway so wide that in places you cannot see either bank. Pink, freshwater 'dolphins' playing around the boat. Endless tracts of dense, impenetrable jungle, with just the odd hut or small settlement, built on stilts along the water's edge. Tiny dugout canoes, barely above the water; flocks of screeching parrots, heron and vultures. As night falls, the total silence and darkness, with it clouds of angry mosquitoes.

The tiny settlement of Maués is stuck in a time warp. The clocks seem to have stopped around the 1920s. But here there is a glimmer of hope. Maués is the centre of the Guarana industry, an industry which is a marriage of tribal wisdom, idealism and modern pharmacology.

Nothing much has changed since the seventeenth century. We found small communities of Indians, two or three families, still producing Guarana in the original way. But this is now an organised industry. Each group collects its own berries, washes them, roasts them in giant clay dishes which they make themselves from river mud, straw and ashes; grinds them with a giant wooden pestle and mortar, rolls the paste into sticks and bakes them over a smoke fire.

This is a true cottage economy, with no factories, no chimneys, no pollution, and above all awareness of the need to preserve the habitat of their main source of income – the Amazon rainforest.

Science is uncovering some of the mysteries of the rainforest plants. Guarana has uses as a tonic and stimulant; it is a mild diuretic and can help treat stomach upsets; it reduces temperature; controls hunger; overcomes fatigue and is a safe mild anti-depressant. According to Professor Accorsi, the herb Lapacho is equally exciting. Long used by the Indians as a treatment for skin problems and scars, it now seems that it may have some anti-cancer action.

As a result of some observational studies at his institute, scientists in America, Japan and Brazil are now working on the chemical actions of this plant. Accorsi stresses that this work is at an early stage, and it could be years before there is a usable body of evidence.

We may not have years left before many of the other plants which could alleviate man's suffering vanish in the face of human greed. People of vision, like Graeme Lewis and his partners in The Rio Trading Company, are fighting to protect the heritage of the rainforest Indians and bring us the benefits of herbs such as Guarana and Lapacho.

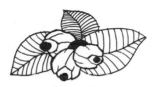

After thirty years spent working in the field of complementary medicine, I have seen the wheel come very nearly full circle. The wisdom of the traditional herbalist is still in use, with drugs like digitalis, curare, quinine and aspirin – albeit synthesised in the chemical laboratory. Modern pharmacology has developed medicines like vincristine – from the Madagascan periwinkle – for the treatment of leukaemia and now we are standing on the brink of amazing discoveries in the rainforest.

The research libraries of the giant pharmaceutical companies bulge with studies of the effects of plant remedies which will never see the light of day. For drug companies to make profits they must have patents and you cannot patent straightforward plant extracts. Unless they can isolate a specific chemical component of a plant and then, by playing molecular roulette with its structure, produce a unique substance, there is no business advantage to be gained from making use of it.

Herbal medicines have served mankind well for thousands of years and now we have the opportunity to open up a whole new world of little-known plant medicines. Sometimes they will replace modern drugs, sometimes they will work alongside them and sometimes they may be used in the general promotion of health and well-being. This book will introduce you to plants you may never have heard of but they are plants that have served the Indians in the rainforest since humans first lived there.

1 *Disaster in the rainforest*

'The tree which moves some to tears of joy is in the eyes of others only a green thing that stands in the way.'
William Blake, 1799

It is almost impossible to open a newspaper or magazine, or to turn on a radio or TV, without being confronted with one of the major environmental or conservation issues of our time. Are we in danger of suffering 'green' burnout? Are we being subjected to a massive environmental hype orchestrated by those with a vested interest in green affairs? Are you getting to the point when you turn over the page or push the off button with a groan, thinking, 'Not another story about the rainforest, the disappearing animals or the endangered species'?

If that is your response, I am saddened but not surprised. Too many of the media stories are high on emotion and low on fact. Too many of those presenting these ideas have a fervour and commitment closer to evangelism than science. Too many of the political pundits are patent hypocrites preaching one gospel for the third world and practising another on their own doorsteps. I've been to the rainforest, journeyed on the waters of the Amazon and its tributaries, flown over the rainforest – which from the air looks like a vast never-ending green carpet which has been ravaged by ravenous hordes of giant moths. I've seen the palls of smoke rising

5

on the horizon for hundreds of miles in every direction and I've
eaten from the communal cooking pots in riverside villages.

When you sit on the banks of the Amazon eating fish cooked
just after being taken from the water and tropical fruits plucked
from the trees, it's hard to believe in the scale of destruction that is
taking place. In the primeval forest, stepping two yards from the
trodden pathways means you are lost in the impenetrable woodlands. In the undamaged regions it seems that the forest is endless
and indestructible, but the sickening jolt of the true scale of the
problem may be just around the next bend.

This is a destruction, a ravaging of our earth's resources, the rape
of a unique and irreplaceable treasure trove, which must be halted.
It seems that the vast majority of us who live in the comfort of the
western world are not concerned enough about the environmental
issues to force our governments to act. I am hopeful that one of
mankind's least attractive emotions will finally come to the rescue.
How many people really care about a handful of forest dwellers
thousands of miles away? Who is really concerned about the effects
on our world environment in the middle of the next century? The
one thing most of mankind has in common is selfishness and in
this book we explore the medical consequences of destroying the
rainforest; we look at the potential benefits to mankind through
the alleviation of pain and illness that we are losing with every acre
of burned and desecrated woodland; we mourn the loss of plants
that just possibly could have cured some forms of cancer, prevented some dreadful disease, relieved some lingering pain.

If enough people are selfish enough to worry about their own
future health and suffering then it will not be too late. I'm not concerned with the reasons why anyone should want to save the rainforest; my only concern is to bring wider notice the thought that in
addition to all the environmental, economic, political and social
reasons there is one more which is often ignored. The medical reason. At the moment you read this page the last traces of a drug as
powerful and life-preserving as quinine, digitalis or curare could be
lost for ever to mankind. I want this thought to disturb you and I
hope that some of the following factual information will make you

more aware of the heritage that we are allowing to vanish for all time.

Mankind's ancestors began life in the trees and, from the time that we descended to the earth, trees have been a source of religious inspiration, shelter, food and fuel. Yet since we put our feet on the ground we have been destroying trees through our own use. If we had never come down from the branches, about half of the world's land mass would still be covered by forests. In earliest times we lived in a harmonious relationship with the woodlands and many early religions worshipped these miracles of nature.

From Confucius to Buddha and from the Vikings to the Druids, to the Garden of Eden where Jews, Christians and Muslims alike recognized the trees of life and knowledge, trees were considered separate and special compared to other plants. But we have somehow managed to develop a love–hate relationship with trees and in the end the trees win. Not by surviving, but by paying back mankind for their destruction. Wherever man abused the forests, disaster followed. Fertile plains became deserts, thriving civilisations vanished, the British colonised far-flung corners of the world to supply wood for naval ships when our own ran out. The ancient Romans and Greeks, iron foundries in Elizabethan England, the demands of war and the demands of people desecrated and decimated the woodlands of the world. Vast areas of once fertile and productive forest land are now our desert inheritance. And it hasn't stopped yet. By cutting down the tropical forests for cattle grazing, beef can be produced at less than half the cost it would be in the US – next time you eat a hamburger, just stop and think that it may have cost the earth two trees.

Imagine yourself taken back in time to the year 1807 BC. You would be one of 3½ million people inhabiting the entire earth, an earth half-covered by primeval forests. A third of those have now vanished for ever. It is horrifying to realise that most of this destruction has happened since the end of the Second World War. The rainforest has suffered particularly badly – around half having been destroyed in this century alone – and Brazil has suffered more than most countries, accounting for around 35% of the world's forest loss every year. In the state of Amazonia we have already seen an area of rainforest the size of Europe disappear. But, tragically, this is only half the picture as twice that amount of the cerrado woodlands has also vanished for all time.

According to the World Wide Fund for Nature (WWF):

At least 400,000 hectares of forest are cleared every week around the world, and this rate of destruction is accelerating alarmingly – an FAO survey shows that deforestation in the tropics almost doubled between 1980 and 1990. If this destruction continues unabated forests will disappear from countries as far apart as Madagascar and Paraguay within the next 20 years. By the year 2025 no large expanses of tropical forests will be left at all, apart from in a few remote parts of Amazonia, Zaire and Papua New Guinea.

Tropical rainforest that would cover the whole of Scotland is destroyed each year and with that destruction goes the loss of the plants that grow there. Although the rainforest now only covers about 6% of the earth's surface, it contains 50% of our plant species, and botanists estimate that by the year 2000 10% of the world's total of 250,000 plants could be extinct. That means the loss of 25,000 species. Since it is statistically likely that 1 in every 125 plants could yield some form of useful medicine, human greed could result in the loss of two hundred plants, any one of which might hold the key to curing a fatal disease.

Industrial sources claim that each lost plant could have a value of $3 billion if it were found to be pharmacologically active. If you think this is just the romantic ramblings of a handful of ecofreaks, then you would be horribly wrong. Historically it is impossible to overemphasise the importance of tropical biological diversity, first to the health of indigenous peoples throughout the tropics, and second to the populations of the rest of the world. The origins of plant-based medicines are shrouded in the mists of time, but the written and precisely documented knowledge of traditional Chinese medicine and Indian ayurvedic medicine is certainly five thousand years old. Even today the importance of traditional plant-based medical systems cannot be overestimated. The World Health Organization is actively encouraging the use and study of traditional healing methods throughout Asia, Africa and Latin America where, for many millions of inhabitants, they are the prime source of treatment.

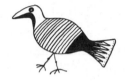

But how relevant is this to someone reading this book in London, New York, Paris, Rome or Sydney? Much more than most people know, is the answer. We all have cause to be grateful for the knowledge and wisdom of tribal medicine men, sages and shamans from as far afield as the rainforest Indians in Brazil to the Aborigines of the Australian outback, from the Bushmen of the Kalahari to the natives of Madagascar. One of the earliest examples is that of cinchona bark from the rainforest of the Andes, the earliest treatment for malaria and the plant from which quinine was subsequently extracted. The drug curare, used as a muscle relaxant in surgery, comes from another Amazonian native plant, the liana. The Madagascan periwinkle has revolutionised the treatment of children with leukaemia – 80% of them now survive. In America the National Cancer Institute believes that there could be two thousand plants in the rainforest with the potential to be useful in the treatment of cancer. An Australian chestnut could produce a drug helpful in the treatment of the HIV virus.

Amongst the giant redwoods and Douglas firs growing in the rainforests of north-western America is a drab, uninteresting tree considered worthless by timber companies. For decades this apparent Cinderella has been grubbed up and burned just to get rid of it. But now the Pacific yew has become linked to a major scientific breakthrough. A chemical isolated from its bark is believed to help in the treatment of breast and ovarian cancers which have not responded to other treatments. Tragically, the Pacific yew is now so scarce that producing sufficient quantities of the drug is a problem. Conservationist Wendell Wood of the Oregon National Resources Council says that he used to plead with the logging firms. 'We would say: "Look guys, the cure for cancer could be out there and you are about to destroy it", and they would say, "Dream on."'

Where else is this happening? It could be in your back yard. Medicines produced from native plants are already worth over $40 billion a year, and plants with the potential to realise drugs worth five times as much are threatened with total eradication every hour of every day. It is tragically true that throughout the world plants are becoming extinct faster than our scientists can study them. Ethnobotanist Dr Steven King has made frequent expeditions to the rainforests in search of more knowledge about the native use of plant medicines. One area which was investigated was the use of plants as anti-fungal remedies, and he found that 69% of the plants used by the tropical peoples his party met have real anti-fungal properties, both as topical skin applications and when taken orally.

He found one plant which was routinely used for fevers, respiratory problems, jaundice, wounds, mouth sores, blindness, malaria, measles, herpes and warts. The unthinking western physician would instantly say, 'Impossible nonsense, how could one medicine be suitable for all these complaints?' But you need look no further than corticosteroid drugs to find that these 'scientific doctors' are quite happy to use the same medication for at least a dozen conditions. King is adamant that we need to approach the skills and traditions of indigenous medicine men with an open mind. He gives a second example of an anti-viral plant with an ethnomedical profile, which is used for diarrhoea, pulmonary problems, cuts, skin irritations, rheumatism, tonsillitis, enhancing fertility, tuberculosis, coughs and flu, haemorrhoids, contraceptives and sore muscles.

This particular plant is now undergoing human clinical trials and shows strong *in-vitro* and *in-vivo* activity against respiratory and flu viruses. The molecule yielded during research, SP-303, cannot be synthesised, and must be produced from natural sources. The clinical trials for SP-303 (Provir) were started in October 1991.

If this is the type of knowledge which we can be privileged to learn from the medicine men, then we must take them extremely seriously. Theirs is an oral tradition passed on from generation to generation. As their numbers decline and as the true native forest dwellers are pushed farther and farther into the jungles, or have their forest homes burned down around them and are forcibly assimilated into other cultures, this knowledge is lost. In fact, as Mark Plotkin of the WWF has said, 'Each time a medicine man dies, it's as if a library has burned down.'

Since Columbus discovered the New World, 95% of South America's Indians have perished. They are victims of our European diseases: victims of conflict and exploitation by the Church, land barons and ruthless governments; victims of forced assimilation; and finally victims of the destruction of their environment.

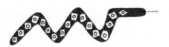

It is not only cattle ranching, the timber industry and mining that is destroying the rainforests. For some forest dwellers themselves there is no alternative to destruction. While the western world basks in affluence and the third world starves, who are we to criticise the poor who, unable to buy agricultural land to feed their families, are forced to clear areas of forest just to subsist? This is poor land whose fruitful life is short, and when it no longer produces sufficient food, it is abandoned and families move even farther into the forests to clear the next patch. Some 150 million people throughout the world survive in this way, eking out a meagre existence at the expense of the earth's great natural resources. The experts calculate that poor people are responsible for 60% of rainforest losses.

Wood is the only available fuel for some two-thirds of the population in the developing world and their relentless foraging for firewood is a major factor in the ever-creeping enlargement of the world's deserts. And whilst we in Britain and the rest of the western world accuse the third-world nations of squandering the earth's resources, and our middle classes rise up *en masse*, join protest movements, wear 'Save the Rainforest' T-shirts, and patronise ecofriendly shops, are we sufficiently without sin to cast the first stone?

History says not, and we haven't even learned from that. We are still importing tropical hardwoods to grace our board-rooms and dining-rooms; we still buy 'added value' products when most of the value is added after those goods leave their country of origin; we are still destroying what little is left of our own ancient forests; we are still ploughing up Sites of Special Scientific Interest; we are still building factories, houses, motorways and railways over land that should be protected; we are still creating our own dust bowls by ripping out hedgerows and monocropping vast areas of cereals; so who are we to criticise?

Countries like Brazil need economic aid and investment from the rest of the world to establish ecologically friendly and sustaining industries within the rainforest. Short-term gains from cattle and timber could be far outweighed in the long term, but the gap between the two systems of generating income has to be bridged with outside help. The revenue from Brazil nuts and rubber tapping, for example, could be four times that generated by cattle ranching, whilst at the same time protecting and enhancing the forest and providing paid employment for large numbers of forest dwellers. If we are to protect the rainforest, it is vital to understand that plants, animals and insects are highly interdependent on each other and that to break the chain is to destroy the forest.

In the twenty years from 1969 to 1989, $700 million of World Bank money was invested in 950 Amazon settlement projects – 631 of them for livestock. According to the Brazilian Planning Ministry, only 16% of the predicted returns were ever achieved. The grazing is so poor that even with different grasses and fertilisers, land that used to support one cow on 2.5 acres, five years later needed 10 acres to support each animal. This is hardly the best use of $700 million, especially when most of it ended up in the pockets of the cattle barons. The whole scheme created very little employment and a great deal of forest destruction.

Schemes that generate local employment, rely on local skills and knowledge and depend on the continuing integrity of the rainforest for their success are possible. Ethnomedicines are certainly one of the keys to the rainforest's survival and companies like Shaman Pharmaceuticals in California and The Rio Trading Company of Brighton, England, are actively engaged in encouraging the wider sale of rainforest medicines, whilst at the same time maintaining the integrity of the forest – essential for the growth of the medicinal plants – and providing paid employment for those that live in the forests.

Graeme Lewis of Rio Trading, and Shaman Pharmaceuticals have the same objectives, to make sure that the local people of the rainforest share in the profits of marketing their plant medicines in the west; to guarantee that the growing, harvesting and processing of the medicines does not endanger the survival of the rainforest, and to ensure that nothing that is done commercially interferes with or puts at risk the natural biodiversity of the forest environment.

Thanks largely to the pioneering work of men like Graeme Lewis, who have brought traditional medicines into the glare of the media and public opinion, phytochemists, ethnobotanists and medical researchers have begun to 'rediscover' some of the homegrown plant medicines. Many Brazilian herbs, for instance, are now widely familiar to doctors and scientists in England, the USA and, particularly, Japan. In some areas these plant-based medicines are even becoming a regular part of orthodox medicine in both general practice and hospitals.

Exotic species like Guarana, Lapacho, Pfaffia, Catuaba, Stevia, Marapuama, Maracuja, Zedoaraia and Boldo are now available in health food stores and pharmacies around the world. Who knows what waits around the corner as more and more scientists start to investigate the folklore of native medicines? We can only hope that the destruction of the forests stops before it is too late. Whether this happens or not depends on each and every one of us. Dealing with the thinning of the ozone layer, atmospheric pollution, global warming and other ecological problems is vital to the survival of our planet, and saving the plants which could hold the key to the relief of much sickness and misery will make our stay on this earth a far better one.

2 Brazil in a Nutshell

Here is a very basic guide to the geography and economics of Brazil.

The geography of Brazil is not directly relevant to an understanding of the medicinal plants of the rainforest, except of course that geography determines climate, and climate determines the habitat in which plants thrive or wither. But this book is a plea for the salvation of the rainforest as much as a book about herbal medicines, so a basic understanding of Brazil and the problems created by its geography is important.

Brazil is the fifth largest country in the world, smaller than only the old Soviet Union, China, Canada and the USA. In fact, it is almost as large as the USA, 8,511,965 sq. km. It comprises almost half of the entire South American continent and, with the exception of Chile and Ecuador, it shares borders with all the other South American countries.

The dimensions are vast, with a north–south dimension of 4,320 km and almost exactly the same from east to west, a land frontier of nearly sixteen thousand km, and an Atlantic coast of 7,400 km. Placed over a map of Europe and Africa, Brazil would stretch from Shannon to beyond the Urals and from Oslo in the north to Timbuctoo in the southern Sahara.

The population of Brazil was 148 million in 1991 – half of the people being aged under 25 – 50% of the population of the whole of South America. The majority of the population live along the strip of coastline occupied by the original Portuguese settlers. In the area from Natal to Recife, Salvador, the states of Minas Gerais, Rio de Janeiro, São Paulo, and Parana there are some ninety million inhabitants; whereas much of the interior areas such as the Mato Grosso and Amazonas has less than one person per square kilometre. The exception to this is the new city of Brasilia, created the federal capital of Brazil on 21 April 1960, which has a population almost at its official maximum of five hundred thousand, and there are some three hundred thousand more people living in shanty towns on the outskirts of the city.

Very little of the land mass of Brazil is level plain, most of it being hilly upland with plateaux and low mountains. The largest of the plains is found in the upper Amazon region in the west of the country and, as you travel downstream, the plain is gradually narrowed by the higher ground on each side. Some of the oldest rock formations on earth, as well as the world's largest lava plateau, are found in the south and this underlying structure is of great interest to geologists.

Broadly speaking, Brazil can be divided into five main areas: the Amazon basin, the River Plate basin, the Guiana Highlands to the north of the Amazon, the Brazilian Highlands south of the Amazon, and the coastal strip. Around 60% of Brazil's total surface area is occupied by the two river basins.

Brazil's climate is surprisingly temperate, in spite of the fact that most of the country lies between the Tropic of Capricorn and the Equator. In the Amazon basin the mean high temperature is between 25° and 26°C. In Rio itself the temperature sits comfortably between 22° and 27°C. and it is only in the dry north-eastern states that temperatures may reach into the low 40s. Brazil's rainfall is surprisingly moderate in most areas except the Amazon basin and rainforest. In general, the total averages between 40 and 60 inches per year, compared with 26 inches in the UK.

Brazil boasts some of the world's great rivers, and these can be divided into three main groups. In the north is the uncomparable Amazon – no matter how many films or photographs you've seen

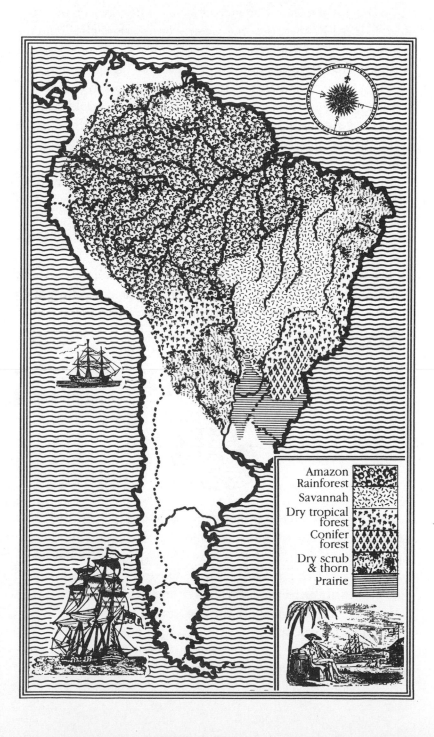

Amazon Rainforest
Savannah
Dry tropical forest
Conifer forest
Dry scrub & thorn
Prairie

of this mighty river, nothing prepares you for its grandeur and vastness. It is fed by the cascading waters coming through mountain peaks, fertile plateaux and huge areas of jungle. The Rio Negro, the Madeira, the Tapajos and the Xingu, the Tocantins and the Araguaia are the tributaries that form the Amazon. But these are not mere streams; anywhere else in the world they would each be considered a great river.

The second group of rivers ends in the Rio de la Plata, where the waters from the Paraná and the Iguazu, fed by some thirty tributaries, arrive after plunging over one of the most spectacular sights in the whole of south America, the Iguacu Falls – 60 feet higher and one and a half times as wide as Niagara – creating columns of spray hundreds of feet high as the waters from the Minas Gerais pour into Argentina.

The final group rises in the plateaux around Brasilia, collecting water from countless tributaries along its thousand-mile length as it flows north forming the great São Francisco River (the largest within Brazil itself) and empties into the sea south of Recife.

Brazilian vegetation varies as much as the landscape and indeed is determined by climate and local geology. The vegetation can be divided into seven main groups.

The *Pine forests*, more common in southern Brazil, are vast areas of coniferous forest whose most famous product is the beautifully marked Paraná pine. Much of it is used for paper, but the best specimens are exported for timber. These pine forests are often a mixture of the tall Paraná pine and a lower level of broad-leaved deciduous trees, one of which is the *Ilex paraguayensis*, used for the preparation of maté tea.

The *selva* is made up of mainly luxuriant broad-leaved evergreens and is found in the Amazon basin and along the Atlantic coast in areas of regular heavy rainfall. The *selva* is crammed with many different types of plants, up to three thousand species in a square mile. The trees grow straight and tall, the branches mingling above forming such a thick canopy that hardly any light reaches through the canopy to the ground beneath.

It is in these north-eastern rainforests that two of the great hardwood trees of South America flourish. One is the huge and beautiful jacaranda tree, used in the manufacture of many pieces of antique furniture found in Brazil; it is similar to mahogany. The other, the Brazil tree, gave the country its name and the rest of world its nuts, although rainforest dwellers tend to eat the fruit and throw away the nuts.

It is this rainforest that pours life-giving oxygen back into the atmosphere which is under such great threat.

Semi-deciduous forest is found where there is slightly less rainfall but where the dry season is very dry. Here grow more broad-leaved trees, mostly evergreen but some are deciduous. The trees do not grow to the size of those in the *selva* and land in these forests is much easier to clear for cultivation. Semi-deciduous forests are found between Natal and Porto Alegre and they cover considerable areas of São Paulo and Minas Gerais. For four hundred years this was the land that supported Brazilian agriculture but, as a result of bad husbandry and little in the way of soil conservation, much of it is now desolate.

The *caatinga* is situated in the dry north-easterly regions, inland from the semi-deciduous forests. Here is found a scrubby, thorny woodland of low-growing and gnarled broad-leaved trees which lose their leaves during the dry periods. Little survives here except goats.

The *campo cerrado* combines savanna with a scrub-like deciduous woodland. This covers vast areas of Brazil's interior south of the Amazon basin rainforest and west of the semi-deciduous forest. *Campo limpo* – areas of pure savanna which develop after many seasons of burning the grass – may be interspersed with patches of uninterrupted woodland.

The *pantanal* combines wet savanna and palm trees. The whole region of the upper Rio Paraguay is covered annually with flood waters but makes excellent grazing during the dry season.

The *prairie* spreads southwards from the state of São Paulo right into Uruguay. Here the *campo cerrado* fades into a tall grass prairie with thickets of trees dotted round the hillsides, and it is here that the Brazilian farmers have traditionally grazed their herds.

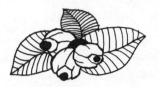

Brazil is a country of enormous geographical and environmental contrasts. It is also a land of immense natural resources and agricultural potential. It is the world's largest producer of coffee and amongst the largest producers of cacao, corn, rice, cotton and beef. Sugar cane is a major crop and also a source of alcohol-based fuel which powers much of the public transport system as well as private cars.

A huge range of valuable minerals and gem stones including gold, diamonds, chrome, nickel, cobalt and high-grade iron ore is present in this country's remarkable geological structure. There are two thousand different varieties of fish in the Amazon alone and thousands more in the other rivers. How tragic it is, therefore, that so little seems to be done to prevent the ravages and rape of the rainforests. Gold prospectors pollute the rivers and poison the inhabitants with mercury residues. The cattle industry razes vast areas of forest to the ground for one or two seasons' grazing and then moves on. The timber moguls decimate the hardwoods and destroy even more of this irreplaceable natural resource.

Brazil and its people, particularly the surviving rainforest Indians, will reap the bitter harvest if the wave of vandalism is allowed to continue. The rest of the world will suffer too as a result of the climatic changes and the destruction of the ozone layer brought about partly through ignorance, and – in today's climate of environmental awareness – to a much greater extent through greed and corruption.

3
A Potted History

The early history of Brazil and its native Indians is important for our knowledge of the medicinal plants that grow there, a knowledge which has survived wars, upheavals, slavery, exploitation and dictatorship. How the Indians learned about the healing properties of the rainforest plants is shrouded in the mists of time, but from the earliest days of European colonisation that knowledge has been gathered together and passed on to the rest of the world. Even in our scientifically sophisticated society, we still have much to learn, and much to gain, from an understanding which began in ancient times, was brought to Europe by the missionary Bettendorf in 1669, and today is being studied, investigated and generally put under the microscope by scientists anxious to unravel the mysteries of the rainforest Indians.

How did it all begin? In 1498 the legendary Vasco da Gama opened up the sea route round the Cape of Good Hope to the spice islands and the Indies. Portugal dispatched a great armada whose purpose was to follow da Gama's route to India under the command of Pedro Alvares Cabral. Despite getting his directions from da Gama in person, Cabral sailed too far to the west and inadvertently arrived on 22 April 1500 at the mainland of South America, which he immediately claimed for Portugal. Originally named Vera Cruz – the true Cross – it soon became Brazil, named after the famous red wood of the pau-brasil tree.

A year later, on 13 May 1501, Amerigo Vespucci left Lisbon to explore the coast of Brazil. As he sailed along the coastline the vastness of this new territory became apparent for the first time. It is Vespucci whom we have to thank for the evocative names, most of which have survived to this day. He christened Rio de Janeiro – river of January – which he first saw on 1 January 1502; the São Francisco river, Cape Santo Agostinho and many other features named after the saint whose day fell on the date of their discovery. Little happened for the next twenty five years, and it was not until 1533 that Brazil was divided into fifteen hereditary fiefdoms which were granted to people of influence. Most of these were a disaster, only two becoming financially successful and stable, and in 1549 King John appointed a governor-general who established his headquarters at the town of Bahia, which survived as the capital of Brazil for 214 years.

With the stability and prosperity that followed, the population began to grow, and agriculture and commerce started to thrive. Soon it became apparent that the local Indian tribes were not a suitable labour force for the new European settlers. They were fiercely independent and always desperate to return to their tribes and families. Forcing them on to the plantations met with little success and at every opportunity they would melt back into the rainforest, where pursuit was highly dangerous and virtually impossible. Desperate for labour, the Portuguese farmers began importing black slaves from Africa and, hideous though this concept is to us, they were laying the foundation for the unique cultural and religious amalgam which forged the fascinating and beguiling character of modern Brazil.

One of the most important influences at this time was the Jesuits. Manuel da Nobrega travelled with the first governor-general to Bahia and laid the foundations for the Jesuits' struggle to protect and convert the Indians. The Jesuits were troubled by the low morals of the European settlers and spared no effort in their endeavours to raise the behavioural standards of the colonists. Nobrega soon built a school to train more missionaries, and as the priests spread throughout Brazil they established small villages for the converted Indians. In 1574 the Jesuits won a royal decree which gave them care and control of the Indians in their villages. This helped stem the tide of Indian slavery as the colonists were only allowed to use tribesmen who were taken in battle and were stopped from rounding up converted Indians *en masse*.

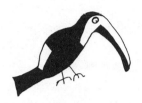

During the next 150 years both the French and the Dutch tried to invade Brazil, but all their efforts ended in dismal failure. Brazil prospered, producing sugar, spices, tobacco, cattle, coffee, gold and precious stones. By 1789 the first rebellion against Portuguese control came and went with the execution of its leaders. The next step on the road to independence came when Napoleon invaded Portugal in 1807. His objective was to make life even more difficult for the English. By attacking Portugal, a long-standing and traditional ally of the British, he would be able to strengthen his blockade of the British Isles.

The king of Portugal, John VI, fled to Brazil together with the entire royal family and boatloads of the nobility, arriving in Rio in March 1808. The king rapidly introduced a string of legal changes and ended the Portuguese commercial monopoly on trade. As a result of free access to all the Brazilian harbours, friendly nations were at last able to buy and sell within the whole of Brazil. Ripples of revolution spread outwards from France and growing discontent in Brazil culminated in an uprising in 1817 which led to the formation of a republic.

This new-found political freedom lasted some ninety days and was finally put down after a considerable struggle, leaving the country in a state of fermenting dissatisfaction which erupted in a full-blown revolution in 1820. On 7 September 1822 Dom Pedro declared the independence of Brazil. The events culminated in the coronation of Dom Pedro as Emperor of Brazil on 1 December. From 1822 to 1889 there was a turbulent period in the country's history. The Brazilian empire suffered civil wars, lawlessness, problems with the army, a war with Paraguay and dreadful economic problems inherited through the slave-based economy of the plantations. In 1831 Brazil abolished the slave trade, but this frightful business continued for more than twenty years before the traffic in slaves was finally ended. Another fifty-seven years of dispute were to pass before the last slaves were finally freed on 13 May 1888. By now there were a number of powerful and disaffected groups within the social structure of the Brazilian empire. The landowners were bitter about lack of compensation for the loss of their slaves; the Church had been antagonised by the way in which some leading dissident bishops were punished; and, most importantly of all, the army had been forbidden by Dom Pedro to have any involvement in politics. On 15 November 1889 a substantial faction of the military establishment revolted, Dom Pedro was forced into abdication and the Republic of Brazil began.

From the beginning of the Republic to the present day, the history of Brazil has been bedevilled by corruption, greed and exploitation. In 1930 the country was ruled by a military junta with Getulio Vargas as dictator. He remained until the army deposed him in 1945. The country was comparatively democratic from 1945 to 1964 but the next five presidents were all from the military, which suppressed all opposition and imposed rigid censorship. There were dreadful stories of torture, murder and extortion. It was not until the election of 1974 that the opposition party made any substantial gains. Since 1930 all governments were guilty of the exploitation of Brazil's mineral resources, fertile plains and huge underpaid labour force. By the 1970s Brazil had outstripped all its neighbours and was the major industrial country of South America, and in 1985 the country held its first democratic election for decades and finally returned to civilian rather than military government. In spite of this, the gap between the rich and poor became greater, inflation ran out of control, and Brazil plummeted into an economic recession of vast proportions with foreign debts that are almost the largest in the world.

In 1989 the government proposed an environmental programme for the Amazon rainforest after worldwide alarm and condemnation over the destruction of this irreplaceable natural resource. Despite this programme, little seems to be changing under the canopy of the rainforest itself. Gold prospectors are poisoning tributaries with mercury, timber companies are raping the forests for short-term commercial gain, and beef producers are burning tens of thousands of acres of woodland to create more grazing for animals destined to provide beefburgers for the West.

Even the democratically elected President Fernando Collor was accused of corruption, impeached and found guilty by both houses of government. His replacement, Itamar Franco, previously vice-president, has an unenviable task. The rate of inflation in 1991 was 440%; the population is growing at around 2% per annum; and the problems of education, health care and crippling international debt appear insoluble.

In spite of all its problems, Brazil is a beautiful country populated by beautiful and friendly people. It is a country of great natural resources and enormous potential, and is likely to be one of the growing tourist areas in coming years. It is a country with more than its fair share of idealists whose commitment to, and love for, their country will hopefully triumph over the historical disasters. During a recent visit to the Amazon region I spent a stimulating and rewarding afternoon with the governor of the Amazonas province – now the mayor of Manaus – Amazonino Mendes. Here is a man with a vision for the future of the rainforest: a man with an acute sense of the importance of preserving and conserving the history and peoples of the rainforests, but at the same time a man with a modern scientific outlook. Some of the Mendes plans for fishing and river-bank cultivation utilise the latest technology and advanced agronomy, but these plans are all designed to protect the environment; provide work, food and income for the inhabitants; and stimulate growth in the local economy without destroying the source of all this potential wealth, the Amazon rainforest.

4 General Information on Plants in Medicine

Since time began, mankind has turned to the world of plants to provide relief from aches and pains and to soothe away the ravages of wind and weather on the skin. There is no inhabited area of our globe that has not yielded some plants from which medicines can be made.

Even in the grave of a Neanderthal man unearthed in Iraq after sixty thousand years, pollen grains from eight different flowers were found scattered around the bones. Seven of these are still in common use today as medicines – for example, the marshmallow for its soothing effects on mucous membranes, the diuretic grape hyacinth, the general tonic yarrow and the *Ephedra* used for centuries in the relief of asthma.

How did our ancestors know which plants to use? Certainly there must have been disasters. Some herbal products at best did not work, and at worst produced a fatal outcome. But there must also have been some instinctive understanding of the properties of plants, similar to that which animals seem to have. You only need to watch your cat or dog to see how they sniff out a particular plant to chew when they are ill. How else could it be possible that tribes of natives as far apart as Fiji, Samoa, India, Trinidad and Vietnam could all use the same remedy, hibiscus tea, for menstrual problems and for the control of fertility? What is even more surprising is that it probably worked. The particular hibiscus they all used has marked anti-oestrogen properties.

The use of medicinal herbs spread throughout the world. Three thousand years before Christ, the Chinese had written down their prescriptions; a thousand years later the Babylonians carved their herbal knowledge on to tablets of stone. From the Ganges to the Nile, information and material were exchanged and traded.

Many new medicines were brought to England by the Roman armies, who never travelled without a supply of plants and seeds. The first thing that their physicians did when a new garrison was established was to plant a herb garden. Plants included mustard and garlic, later to become staples of British herbalists.

The Welsh druids, the monks and traditional folklore all added to our body of information, and herbal medicine flourished up to the early twentieth century. It was the great Prussian biochemist Paul Ehrlich who sounded the death knell with his 'magic bullets' concept of 'a pill for every ill'. And from then on, the pharmaceutical industry was on the path to domination of the entire drug scene.

There can be no denying that many drugs have made untold contributions to the welfare and survival of sick people: antibiotics, pain-killers, anti-inflammatories and all the rest which no sane person would wish the world to be without. But sadly, their efficacy has caused many people to reject the entire field of herbal medicine, regarding it as mere folklore and mumbo jumbo. This is in spite of the fact that many of the major 'new' drugs were derived from plant material. Even now, some 25% of prescriptions contain at least one important ingredient from the herbal world. Digoxin, quinine, morphine, atropine, codeine, ephedrine and vincristine are just some of these in every day use.

Quack or cure?

With a few notable exceptions like belladonna and some other poisons, herbal medicines are safe and effective. Yet the majority of doctors dismiss these gifts from nature as 'quack' cures. They regard reports of the properties of plant preparations as little more than old wives' tales, and continue to prescribe larger and larger quantities of drugs which often have side-effects. The period from the 1950s to the 1990s will go down in medical history as the time of a great epidemic: an epidemic caused not by bacteria, viruses, environmental pollution or holes in the ozone layer, but by the doctors themselves. This is an epidemic that accounts for one in five of patients that fill hospital beds, an epidemic of ill-health caused by the side-effects of drugs used to treat ill-health. This is the epidemic of iatrogenic disease – the name given to illnesses caused by treatments for other illnesses.

There are many situations in which the gentler action of herbs, with the relative lack of unwanted counter-effects, would be appropriate. The public has become uneasy about the over-use of powerful drugs, and is turning to the plant world for the treatment of minor ailments.

There is now a revolution going on, concerned with the scientific investigation of herbal preparations. Research is now able to

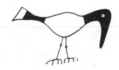

prove just how often the old wives were right and, in many cases, bears out the wisdom of the ancient herbalists.

It may have surprised you to discover that the origins of modern medicine, with its heavy reliance on drug prescriptions to treat specific diseases, lie in herbalism. Just as the medical herbalist has at his or her disposal a large number of drugs from plant and plant material, so has today's conventional allopathic doctor. A surprising proportion of the drugs that today's doctors prescribe are little different from those handed out in the nineteenth century, and some of the best modern drugs are purified products of herbs.

Plant power

Some very well-known drugs have been refined from plants and are in worldwide use. Digitoxin from the foxglove (*Digitalis purpurea*) and digoxin from the closely related *D. lanata* are both used as cardiotonics and to treat heart failure. Atropine from deadly nightshade (*Atropa belladona*) is used to dilate the pupil (in eye surgery, for example). Morphine from the opium poppy (*Papaver somniferum*) is a powerful painkiller; quinine from *Cinchona officinalis* is used to treat malaria. Perhaps the best known of all is aspirin. Aspirin was originally synthesised from salicylic acid obtained from the white willow (*Salix alba*). It should be added in this context that some of the more dangerous and well-known modern drugs are not derived from herbs or plants but are manufactured synthetics. Valium and sleeping tablets are examples. It is these drugs that tend to cause the most side-effects.

How safe are plants?

Herbal treatments have been in use for thousands of years. Herbal remedies have been passed down the generations, first by word of mouth and then in illustrated herbals. Their drug trials, therefore, have been carried out on previous populations. With today's drugs, new products have to be used in trials first on animals, then on human volunteers, and finally are released on the market. It is not unusual for a so-called wonder drug to be withdrawn comparatively quickly after its release because of unsuspected side-effects. Certainly, there are plants which are poisonous or which cause undesirable side-effects, but the herbalist has very extensive trials and records at his or her disposal enabling him or her to prescribe safely. While herbalists are able to prescribe drugs with no harmful side-effects, it may be that their drugs are not as powerful as those prescribed by allopathic doctors.

The whole story

A crucial difference between medical herbalists and today's orthodox doctors is that the herbalist looks at the patient as a whole,
while conventional doctors look for symptoms which enable them
to diagnose and treat diseases. They see the patient as a disease carrier, whereas the herbalist regards the patient as a diseased person
requiring holistic treatment.

Secondly, the medical herbalist is using medicines made from
the original plant – whether the root, bark, stem, leaf, flower, seed
or the entire plant is used, all the constituents present in the original material are found in the remedy. Modern medicine extracts
what it believes to be the single active principle from the plant and
uses that in isolation or possibly synthesises it in the laboratory.

Herbal medicine involves use of the whole plant, the combination of all its constituents, and these work together in natural harmony to exert specific therapeutic effects on the body. Any plant
contains a number of constituents; these may include alkaloids,
glycosides, tannins, gums, resins, trace minerals, essential oils,
antibiotic substances and hormone precursors. Each of these has a
function and may reinforce, support or control the action of the
others. Herbal practitioners are strongly opposed to the principle of
isolating one constituent, knowing from experience that the greatest value is in the sum of all the constituents. Furthermore, the safety and efficacy of the whole plant is far greater than that of the isolated constituents. The gentle action of these remedies is effective,
safe and in harmony with the body's therapeutic needs. This is
especially well illustrated in the case of Guarana since, as will be
explained elsewhere in the book, it is the complex actions of the
various constituents of the plant that produce its unique actions on
the body. These are actions that would be either extreme or non-
existent if the individual chemical components of Guarana were
administered as separate specific drugs.

Plant interaction

One constituent of a plant may either negate a potential undesirable side-effect of another of its constituents or potentiate the effect of a third constituent (a process known as *synergism*). This makes it desirable, herbalists believe, to use whole plants rather than only the active substances. Furthermore, and this is central to the skill of medical herbalism, plants can interact with each other to produce either a different, a better or a worse remedy.

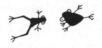

Several different plant extracts may be contained in one preparation with the intention that each will produce its specific effect to accomplish a beneficial combined effect. Herbal combination therapy, which is clearly complex, is the rule rather than the exception for medical herbalists and that is why you should seek a reputable and qualified practitioner. The practice of medical herbalism requires diagnostic skills as well as a vast knowledge of the herbal pharmacopoeia and a detailed understanding of the way in which herbal medicines may interact with one other.

The National Institute of Medical Herbalists is the leading organisation in the UK. It runs long-term intensive training courses and publishes a register of its qualified members. If you are seeking professional advice as opposed to using simple herbals for minor ailments, then look for the letters MNIMH as your assurance of proper training and safe care. In the USA contact the American Botanical Council, Austin, Texas.

Herbal renaissance

The resurgence of interest in herbalism today has taken place partly in line with an increasing demand for natural foods and natural remedies and a growing distrust of synthetics in all fields; and partly as a result of increased scientific research on plants themselves.

There are an estimated 250,000 plant species in the world. While only a small percentage has been evaluated so far, this area of research is growing. The World Health Organization, in its quest to provide adequate medical care for all by the year 2000, is investigating and supporting traditional herbal medicines in third-world countries. Studies are being carried out on the traditional herbs used in these countries and people are being encouraged to share knowledge and to undertake training. China is also directing further research into herbal medicine.

The experts believe strongly that this research will pay dividends in the end, although there is still a hard core of resistance to herbal medicines. According to Norman Farnsworth, arguably the world's leading pharmacognosist, who is professor of pharmacognosy and senior university scholar at the University of Illinois, Chicago:

> There are 121 prescription drugs in use today in many different countries in the world that come from only 90 species of plants. Of those, 74% came from following up the claims of native folklore. There are 250,000 species of plant on the planet. A logical person would have to say there are a lot more jackpots out there.

It is certainly true that some of the drug company research designed to evaluate medicinal plants has been expensive and ineffective. Farnsworth suggests that the sceptical attitudes prevalent in the scientific establishment conducting this research are hardly likely to produce exciting results.

Barbara Griggs, in her definitive and heavily researched history of herbal medicine, *Green Pharmacy*, illustrates that this scepticism was still prevalent in the 1960s when she quotes from the *American Journal of Pharmacy*:

> one thing hasn't changed in the last 25 years. Back in 1942 many scientists considered plant drugs the remnant of a dark age, from which we would soon be liberated by organic synthesis ... and today very much the same attitude prevails.

Almost thirty years on little has changed for the better. The

World Health Organization urges greater use and more study of native plant remedies whilst governments impose stricter and stricter legislation and drug companies continue their search for magic bullets.

The regular use of herbal teas and tisanes to replace coffee, tea and other social drinks; in cooking; and in the early stages of illness does much to promote good health. A simple infusion of elderflower (*Sambucus nigra*) and peppermint (*Mentha x piperita*) taken hot in the first hours of a cold or influenza has been found to disperse the illness quickly. If combined with abundant amounts of fresh garlic or tablets made from whole crushed garlic taken each night during the winter, recurrent colds and catarrh, with their potential complications – such as bronchitis – can become a thing of the past.

The stresses of modern life are responsible for an alarming increase in nervous problems such as depression, anxiety and insomnia – and a resultant dependence on anti-depressants, tranquillisers and sleeping tablets. There are many calming herbal treatments, known as nervines, which have a gentle sedative action on the nervous system, such as skullcap (*Scutellaria lateriflora*), valerian (*Valeriana officinalis*), vervain (*Verbena officinalis*) and balm (*Melissa officinalis*). These can be taken regularly or occasionally without the hazard of withdrawal symptoms. Stress-related disorders can also be treated with Bach remedies, created by Dr Edward Bach who practised from the 1910s until his death in 1936. These are plant tinctures given in homoeopathic dosages to treat negative moods and states of mind.

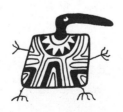

Hypertension and angina, both often stress-related, can respond to herbal treatments. Neither is a suitable condition for self-treatment, but it does help to take tisanes of lime blossom (*Tilia cordata*) or chamomile flowers (*Chamamaelum nobile*) in place of coffee and tea, which are both stimulants. They will also reinforce hypotensive remedies intended to help lower the blood-pressure.

An extensive range of herbs is available to treat migraine, but the causes should be assessed before specific remedies are taken. 'The herbal remedy which has gained the most popular renown recently is feverfew (*Chrysanthemum parthenium*), recommended over four hundred years ago for vertigo and used today for the relief of migraine. Taken as tablets, or using a couple of fresh leaves in a sandwich – chewed on their own they can cause mouth ulcers – feverfew will often bring a rapid end to a migraine attack. Some sufferers find that a daily dose will even prevent their migraine from developing. Feverfew is easy to grow in the garden or in a large pot on the windowsill.

The herbalist's vocabulary

Many of the descriptions of herbal treatments are the same as those used by conventional doctors: for example, anti-spasmodic, expectorant, diuretic, emetic, stimulant. Some, however, are used only rarely by other types of practitioners:

*   **carminative** – relieves flatulence and colic
*   **cholagogue** – helps or stimulates the release of bile from the gallbladder
*   **demulcent** – soothing substance for the skin
*   **emenagogue** – stimulates menstruation
*   **emollient** – used internally to soothe membranes or on the skin to soften
*   **nervine** – calming
*   **vulnerary** – used to treat and heal wounds.

Alternative names for herbalism that you may come across are eclectic medicine, plant healing, physiomedicalism, medical herbalism, herbology, botanic medicine and phytotherapy.

From our Neanderthal man in his flowerstrewn grave to primitive jungle tribes and on to the modern herbal medicine of the twentieth century, the history of plants in the treatment of disease is filled with larger than life figures. The Chinese herbalist Shen Nung had a list of nearly four hundred plant medicines in 2800 BC. In ancient Babylon stone carvings reveal fascinating herbal information from the court of King Hammurabi – there are prescriptions involving plants such as mint, licorice and henbane, all used thousands of years ago for the same purposes as they are today.

From the Nile to the Ganges we find familiar names amongst herbal medicines that were traded between nations more than a thousand years before the birth of Christ: linseeds, the basis for many cough remedies; the white poppy, opium's source; juniper; garlic; and even cannabis, prized for its soothing properties. By the fourth century BC the Greeks possessed the earliest of herbals listing plants and their uses.

How sad it is that King Alfred is mainly remembered for burning the cakes. During the last period of his reign he became very interested in medicine and on his specific instructions some of the great European medical literature was translated into English and made widely available. As a result of Alfred's enthusiasm there was a much greater knowledge of plants in Britain than in the rest of Europe. There were nearly three times as many plants named in English, together with their uses, as were listed by our neighbours at that time.

Centuries later it must be time for much closer co-operation between modern scientific medicine and traditional medical herbalism. Throughout history we have tended to throw away the old in favour of the new – the wheel was adopted instead of the sledge, the printed newspaper replaced the town crier, the internal combustion engine was used instead of the horse. Nowhere have these changes been more dramatic than in modern medicine. But in discarding the old are we in danger of throwing out the baby with the bathwater? The incredible progress of medical technology has revolutionised both diagnosis and treatment. We have the ability to make coronary by-pass surgery a routine procedure; there have been amazing advances in diagnostic techniques with the advent of the CAT scan, MRI and ultrasound scans; and key-hole microsurgery allows patients to be treated as day cases and go back to work within the week when ten years ago they might have spent two weeks in hospital and had two months off work for the same operation.

For a while it seemed as though we had conquered some of the worst diseases that afflict our planet – smallpox, tuberculosis, leprosy and polio – but, in spite of the fact that the life expectancy of a child born today is thirty years more than that of a child born in 1900, there are some storm clouds gathering on the horizon of orthodox medicine. There are fears of smallpox returning, there are resistant strains of tuberculosis ravaging some communities in America, the incidence of many forms of cancer is on the increase. Looked at dispassionately, much of the improvement in public health is due more to improvements in public hygiene than to improvements in medicine. Prince Albert was right when he complained about the drainage and sewage systems in London, so right in fact that typhoid, linked to poor public hygiene, killed him at an early age, together with hundreds of thousands of Queen Victoria's loyal subjects.

Why, in this era of huge hospitals, multi-national drug companies and high-tech medicine, are so many people turning towards alternative medicine, even in countries such as the UK where free health care is available to all? I believe that there are three answers.

- First, because the public is more and more concerned about the side-effects linked to many pharmaceutical preparations.
- Second, because medicine has conspicuously failed to deal with many of the chronic, disruptive, but non life-threatening problems which beset an ever-ageing population.
- Third, because patients are no longer content to give up total

control of their health care to the autocrats of the medical profession. Nor are they prepared to continue to be treated as a collection of symptoms rather than as individual human beings.

According to Ara H. Der Marderosian, professor of pharmacognosy and medicinal chemistry at the Philadelphia College of Pharmacy and Science:

> At least 25% of all prescription drugs sold contain some plant component and, until the advent of biotechnology, only seven major drugs could be synthesised more cheaply than they could be gathered ... It is obvious that if modern medicine were to pay more attention to the fact that people use herbs, both could benefit enormously.

The NHS would benefit through a far cheaper drugs bill, the costs of treating much of the iatrogenic disease would be less, and the patients would benefit as a result of fewer side-effects and more 'user-friendly' medicaments.

Many of the modern products of the pharmaceutical industry make the difference between life and death, but before prescribing any medicine there is a risk–benefit equation to be balanced. It is undeniable that the benefits frequently far outweigh the risks involved in treating serious illness; after all, the ultimate risk is that the patient will die without treatment. But, sadly, there is now a huge body of evidence which tells us that many prescription medicines are used as sledgehammers to crack small nuts and that the risks of medication frequently outweigh the benefits. This book is a plea for a wider prescription of gentler treatment, a wider use of plant medicines and a wider scientific outlook on the world which we inhabit.

New scientific discoveries abound in the field of plant medicine, but nowhere is there a larger untapped source of dramatic potential than in the plant world of the Amazon rainforest. This book is dedicated to the rainforest Indians and their extraordinary cultural traditions. Our so-called civilization has a great deal to learn from them about the use of plants as medicines. They may not have the scientific understanding about how or why they work, but they surely know that they do work. By expanding our scientific knowledge of rainforest medicines we should not only benefit the inhabitants of of our western world but also create much wider benefits. By encouraging the cultivation and use of native plants within the rainforest and consequently creating a cottage economy which provides income and desperately needed foreign currency, we support an industry which will only survive if the forest remains intact. Hopefully this book may go some way to opening new uses for the Amazon rainforest and so provide yet one more reason for halting the massive destruction of forest lands through cattle production and the appalling pollution of waterways in the search for gold.

5
Guarana

Of all the medicinal plants of the Brazilian rainforest, the best known is Guarana or, to give it its proper name, *Paullinia cupana*. Other popular names for this plant are Brazilian cocoa and Guarana bread. It has been known to the rainforest Indians since time immemorial and found its way to Europe through the early explorers in the latter part of the seventeenth century. As early as 1893 *Everybody's Pocket Cyclopaedia*, published by Saxon and Co., carried this note:

> In four and a half years POCKET CYCLOPAEDIA has spread itself in this country (outside the great range of its American publication) to the extent of 560,000 copies. It is our continuous effort to render the book trustworthy and abreast of the latest information, and so in these and all respects more and more worthy of such handsome appreciation

In the health section of the *Cyclopaedia* there is an entry that reads as follows:

> Megrim, or Sick Headache. – There are several varieties of megrim, the best known forms being hemicrania, blind headache, and bilious headache. This complaint occurs more commonly in women than in men, the first attack often making its appearance about the age of ten. The

seizures usually come on once or twice a month, and may last three or four days, totally incapacitating the patient from exertion of any kind. Sometimes they are accompanied by attacks of double vision, and sometimes they terminate with a sharp bout of sickness. Not infrequently they are associated with neuralgia, and many remedies which are recommended for megrim are applicable to the treatment of nerve pain. Susceptibility to attacks depends very much on the condition of the general health. The complaint occurs much more frequently when the patient is underfed, takes too little exertion, or suffers from constipation. One of the best remedies for this complaint is Guarana or Brazilian Cocoa, which should be given in five-grain doses, three times a day.

A Modern Herbal by Mrs M. Grieve and Mrs C. F. Leyel – subtitled *The Medicinal, Culinary, Cosmetic and Economic Properties, Cultivation and Folklore of Herbs, Grasses, Fungi, Shrubs and Trees with all their modern scientific uses* and originally published in 1931, was the first comprehensive encyclopaedia of herbs since the days of Culpeper. The *Herbal* describes Guarana as a:

nervine, tonic, stimulant, aphrodisiac and febrifuge ... The tannin it contains is useful for mild forms of diarrhoea and its chief use in Europe and America is for headache ... It is a gentle excitant and serviceable where the brain is irritated or depressed by mental exertion, or where there is fatigue or exhaustion from hot weather ... Its benefit is for nervous headache or the distress that accompanies menstruation or exhaustion following dissipation ... It is used by the Indians for bowel complaints.

There is a growing body of modern scientific evidence to show that Guarana is indeed a valuable therapeutic plant possessing considerable benefits and producing virtually no side-effects. It has a long history of traditional use by the rainforest Indians and was enthusiastically adopted by most of the early European visitors to the Amazon basin. In addition it was a valuable source of commerce. As early as 1819 the botanist von Martius found a bustling business transporting Guarana from Maués as far afield as Bolivia and the Mato Grosso. As we shall see, today that commerce is even more important, not only because Guarana is a valuable export commodity and hard currency earner for Brazil, but because it is a cash crop both for the primitive rainforest families producing it as tradition dictates and for the larger plantations which function on a more European-style business footing.

First discovered by the Maués-Saterés tribe, Guarana has been used for thousands of years as a tonic and stimulant. So valuable was it to the tribesmen that this plant was a form of currency throughout the rainforests. The earliest reports of the value of Guarana came from a missionary called Bettendorf. The Maués-Saterés were by far the sturdiest and healthiest tribe that he found during his travels in the forest. In 1669 he wrote of the way in which the Indians used the plant to help them cope with the extreme heat, to carry them through long journeys, to suppress the appetite and to relieve headaches, fevers and cramp.

This extraordinary plant gets its name from a native word which means 'secret eyes'. If you are ever fortunate enough to see it growing you will know why. The fruit of this luxuriant shrub hangs in great bunches, like bright red grapes. The red pods split to reveal chestnut-brown seeds with a round white middle. As you walk in the forest they are like a million eyes staring out at you.

For the Maués-Saterés Indians Guarana has been more than just a useful food and medicine for thousands of years. To them it is seen as a gift from the gods. Its cultivation, production and use are imbued with ancient myths and rituals. For the Indians its medicinal value and the way in which this plant stimulates the brain and keeps the body active and vital is nothing less than a miracle. To survive in the hot, humid and hostile environment where they live, alertness and vigour are essential. It is their dependence on Guarana which they believe helps them in their continuing battle against the jungle.

Indian folklore, handed down the tribe from generation to

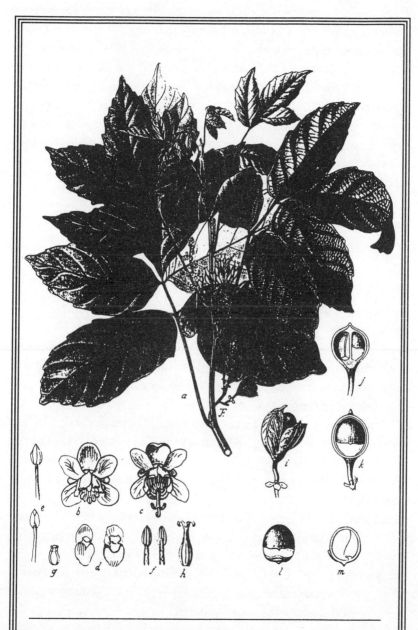

Paullinia cupana, Sapindaceae. vulg. Guarana

generation of camp-fire storytellers, explains the origins of Guarana. Back in the mists of time a boy was born into the tribe. He was no ordinary child, but was gifted beyond their experience – so gifted that he aroused the jealousy of the forest spirits, one of who slew this child in the depths of the forest. The body of the prodigy was carried ceremoniously back to his village home and embalmed, but his eyes were buried in the soil of the forest. From that very spot the vine of the Guarana sprang from the ground, bringing the gifts of eternal watchfulness and constant alertness – gifts which endow mankind with the only answers to the problems of surviving the rigours and dangers of life in the Brazilian rainforest.

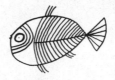

I drove in an open truck, during a tropical thunderstorm, through one of the largest plantations in the Amazon. There the seeds are harvested and processed as they have been for generations. First they are soaked to remove the outer husks; then they are washed, dried, crushed and roasted over wood fires. The next step is to bake them into sticks of hard 'bread' which are easy to carry.

Traditionally, the day starts with a cup of Guarana tea. It is made by grating the end of a bread-stick into boiling water. The grater is the bone-hard, rough palate of an Amazonian fish, the pirarucu. I ate the fish, which was wonderful, and shared the tea with the local Indians.

As well as producing this traditional form of the herb, more convenient products such as capsules and dry powder are made for export all over South America, and now even to Great Britain, the USA and the rest of the world. The national soft drink in Brazil is not the universal 'Coke', but one made from the Guarana seed.

The local Indians also use Guarana paste to make decorative items. They shape it into figures of men, animals, plants, groups of people, and even into tableaux of village life. The models are often decorated with paints made from local natural dyes and minerals, and the finished objects abound with the vitality and humour of these delightful people. The traditional value of these objects far outweighs their simple beauty. Made as they are from one of the Indians' most precious medicines and foods, they take on a spiritual, almost religious importance.

So, what is it that makes this plant so valuable to man?

The Guarana plant is a miracle of evolution. It survived by climbing the giant trees of the Amazon jungle in order to reach the sun. But the Indians managed to tame this vigorous creeper and over the centuries have cultivated it into a robust energetic shrub. They rescued it from the forest and planted it in village clearings. As it thrived they were able to harvest its valuable crop of seeds without scaling the massive native trees in order to reach the canopy, sometimes almost two hundred feet from the ground.

The Guarana now thrives, flowers and gives up its seeds all over the Amazon region. Local residents even grow it in their back gardens. This 'elixir of eternal youth', as the Indians know it, presents the scientists with a paradox. The natives use it for a number of opposite reasons: it increases physical stamina and reduces the appetite; it is an effective treatment for diarrhoea and equally good for constipation; it improves tolerance to heat and humidity and can be a cooling refreshing drink.

The small but growing town of Maués is the centre of the Guarana industry. The boats that tie up along the river bank await their cargoes of local people, chickens, bicycles – and 80% of the world's Guarana production, which they handle. Chalk-written signs give you the destination, departure date and time, give or take a few days and several hours. The Maué-Acu river is a tributary of the great Amazon and it is three to four days journey to Manaus, the destination for most of the Guarana production. From there trains of barges travel downriver to the major sea port of Belém.

During the nineteenth century the miraculous powers attributed to Guarana by the Indians were investigated by the leading scientists of the day, such as the French chemist Vereg and the German von Martius. In 1941 the Brazilian Ministry of Agriculture published a work by Frederico Schmidt in which he describes Guarana tea as having a bitter taste and being astringent, with properties of interest to the human metabolic system.

According to the seventeenth-century missionary, Joao Felipe Bettendorf – the first European to uncover the wonders of Guarana – the Guarana fruit is dried, after which:

> It is stamped on to make a ball which the Indians value as much as the whites value their gold. The fruit is broken open with a small stone and the Indians mix the water in a small gourd. This drink is so powerful that while hunting, the Indians do not feel hunger from one day to the next. The drink also makes one urinate, cures fevers, headaches and cramps.

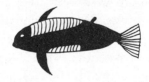

There is a strict ritual for the traditional preparation of Guarana. This is followed closely by the small groups of forest dwellers who now make their living all around the Maués region. The harvest begins when the first fruit is visible. The fruit is shelled by hand and left to soak for two days in water to soften the pulp.

The softened seeds are then heaped into closed fibre baskets like giant tea strainers and washed in the river to remove the pulp. I stood with a husband and wife as they heaved the baskets in and out of the flowing water, while their children kept a sharp eye out for the alligators.

The seeds are then poured into a large dish about six feet across and nine inches deep, made from the local river-bank clay. The dish is built, into supports over a fireplace fuelled by wood. The fire is built up gradually and as the seeds dry out they are stirred with a wooden paddle. By now the fire is raging, the seeds are roasting until they pop and the sweat is pouring from the man with the paddle. When all that day's seeds are roasted, they are removed from the clay dish until it has cooled a little. Then the seeds are replaced in the dish and left overnight to lose any moisture still remaining.

The next morning the roasted seeds are put into a coarse sack made from jute. Banging the sack on the ground shucks off the thin dried skin left on the seeds. The skins are sieved out and then it is time to make the paste. A kilo of seeds is mixed with twenty spoonsful of water – the scales I saw were a primitive balance with two pans, one for the seeds, the other with a 500 g bag of rice on it – and pounded in a home-made pestle and mortar. Once the paste is the right consistency, it is time for the women and children to take over. The paste is rolled into a cigar-like sausage about nine inches long and just over an inch thick.

The final stage of this time-honoured ritual production is the smoking. The sticks of Guarana are smoked to dry them and darken their colour. This is done in a specially constructed smoke house, a small cabin with a thatched roof. Inside there are shelves made from the local reeds. The Guarana sticks are first stacked on the bottom shelves, gradually moving up the building until they reach the top. The smoke is generated by a fire of local green wood on the floor of the cabin, which is kept going night and day. By the end of smoking the sticks are rock hard and they will keep for a whole year or more if they are in a dry place. It is typical of these locally produced Guarana sticks that there will be the occasional uncrushed seed and variations in consistency. These irregularities add to the value as they show that the sticks have been made by the traditional methods and not in the new commercial plants.

The Brazilian government, in spite of its many shortcomings over the years, has become aware of the importance of the local production of Guarana by traditional methods by the indigenous inhabitants of the rainforest. FUNAI (the National Indian Foundation) has set up a number of projects since 1980 to improve the local production of Guarana. Under the direction of the FUNAI regional authority in Manaus there are now many co-operatives in the reservations where Guarana plantations have been established and the traditional methods of production encouraged. The proceeds go to the rainforest Indians.

Industrial production of Guarana also takes place on a large scale. The two major brewing companies, Brahma and Antarctica, are the largest producers of Brazil's national drink, a sweet fizzy beverage made with Guarana extract. I visited the Antarctica plantation – the size of Guernsey – where huge amounts of Guarana concentrate are produced for the soft drink industry. Obviously the cultivation, harvesting and production are highly mechanised here, though the main difference is in the fact that all the by-products are sold for other commercial purposes. The basic principles remain the same, though in practice each stage is performed by machines instead of men. Most of the concentrate produced here is to supply the nationwide domestic market for Guarana drinks. But a fair proportion is exported to other South American countries where the beverage is equally popular. Today you can drink it in North America, Europe, the UK, and most other places too.

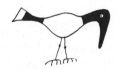

Each December the fascinating riverside town of Maués hosts the annual Guarana Festival, where the local people celebrate their 'gift from the gods'. Travellers from around the world now join in these celebrations and enjoy, as I did, a meal on the white sand lapped by the dark waters of the Maué-Acu river. The throbbing rhythms of the lambada roll across the beaches as local bands entice the revellers to dance under the sun. The history of Guarana is re-enacted by recounting the legends of the past, whilst the future looks all the better for the worldwide interest in this remarkable plant.

One of the main constituents of Guarana is a chemical called guaranine. This is similar in structure to caffeine, which explains its tonic and stimulating effects. There have been attempts to isolate the active principle and use it as a medicine. But, as so often happens, the native wisdom has been proved right. The Indians only ever use the whole seed and this works without side-effects. Though the caffeine-like properties are present, in combination with the other ingredients in the plant they have a gentle and sustained effect.

The tannin content is relatively high too, and this explains why Guarana is so good for the treatment of diarrhoea and digestive problems. What is more, there are potent saponins, similar to those found in Ginseng. It is these that balance the stimulation produced by the guaranine. I am certain that Guarana tea is a good substitute for tea and coffee. It will provide that lift which we have come to expect, but in a much gentler and longer-lasting way. It could be useful for those who need to avoid caffeine and those with migraine or high blood-pressure who feel like a light stimulant at sometime during the day.

The Indians say that Guarana prevents and combats fatigue, stimulates brain function, aids concentration, relieves headache and menstrual pain, helps the body get rid of water, combats the discomfort of extreme heat, speeds recovery after illness and reduces appetite.

So, who can benefit from these 'secret eyes' from the jungle? Anyone under stress or pressure – of examinations, interviews, work or social functions. And it can be used at times of illness, during convalescence or after childbirth. Athletes, walkers, climbers, cyclists – anyone needing to maintain high levels of energy over extended periods when it might not be practical or possible to consume normal food – will find it useful.

One highly disturbing trend in the pattern of health and disease has emerged and has become a problem of growing magnitude since the mid-1980s. This is the ever-increasing number of patients consulting their doctors because of feelings of exhaustion and fatigue, to such an extent that this is now the commonest reason for patients to visit their family doctor. Chronic fatigue is a common symptom of depression and it is most unfortunate that all too often these poor patients are hustled out of the surgery with nothing more than a prescription for anti-depressants – after all, writing a prescription is the quickest way of ending the consultation.

Certainly some of these patients will be suffering from clinical depression, but the vast majority are not. Even when they do get depressed, that depression may well be the result of some underlying problem. Who would not feel depressed after weeks or months of being too tired to get up and shave in the morning, or too exhausted to make breakfast for the children, or so utterly worn out that the effort of getting dressed is too daunting even to contemplate? In situations like these the depression is the effect and not the cause of the patient's condition.

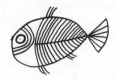

Before exploring some of the scientific evidence for the value of Guarana, let me tell you about coping with the modern epidemic of fatigue and how Guarana has enabled me to make an enormous difference to many of my patients.

ME, TAT and SAD

ME – myalgic encephalomyelitis, post-viral fatigue syndrome or chronic fatigue syndrome, sometimes derogatively known as 'yuppie flu'; TAT – tired all the time syndrome; and SAD – seasonal affective disorder – are three very separate problems with one common factor. Together with all the other symptoms which are involved in these conditions, virtually all sufferers from any of them have a desperate shortage of energy and stamina.

Millions of people wake up tired every morning wondering how they will survive the coming day. Tiredness is the commonest symptom complained of and more than a third of the population suffers from it at any one time throughout the developed world.

Everyone feels tired sometimes. Late nights, a bad day at work, family problems, travel frazzle, or just the lack of a break – all these can wear you down. But chronic fatigue leaves you listless, lacking in energy and waking exhausted every day. If this sounds familar and you feel constantly too tired to cope, then this action plan to boost your energy will help you back to vitality and bring back your zest for life.

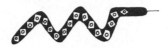

In the past few years the number of patients coming through my surgery with severe fatigue problems such as ME and the newly named TAT and SAD has risen dramatically. Even with these severe problems the traditional principles of Naturopathy have produced gratifying results. My action plan is one which helps the body to help itself into a better state of health and vitality, but at the same time does nothing to interfere with the vital forces of nature.

One of the most dramatic aids to the treatment of severe fatigue is the magical Brazilian herb Guarana, which I have added to this beat-fatigue regime since my first eye-opening visit to the Brazilian rainforest.

Constant fatigue may be caused by underlying medical conditions. Anaemia, especially in menstruating women; thyroid, hormone and heart problems; chronic pain; viral infections; and even allergy may be the cause. If you are permanently tired you must seek professional help in order to exclude underlying disease. Even if there is a medical reason for your condition you can still follow this action plan together with any other prescribed treatment.

1.   *Avoid the energy robbers*

These are your hidden enemies. Beware of the things that rob your body of what little energy you have.

Refined carbohydrates like sugar, white flour, cakes, biscuits, sweets and puddings. Excessive fats, especially the hidden fats in processed and fast foods. Alcohol, which destroys vitamins C and B. Caffeine in tea, coffee, chocolate and cola drinks – they interfere with your uptake of iron. Nicotine, which interferes with vitamin B absorption and reduces oxygen in the blood. High-energy drinks, which are rich in glucose and may give you an instant lift but do you no good at all in the long term.

2. Diet

If you are always tired, then shopping, cooking and planning meals becomes impossible. Snacking on poor-quality foods makes the problem worse and you become locked into a vicious circle of exhaustion, poor food and more exhaustion.

Easily digested and nutritious superfoods are what you need – almonds, apricots, bananas, broccoli, spinach, brown rice, sesame and sunflower seeds, wholewheat bread, potatoes, pasta, porridge, eggs, fish, poultry, lean meat and low fat dairy products, together with masses of fresh fruit and salads.

There are four golden rules for your energy eating plan.

• Eat regularly and little and often. Never go more than three hours without food. This keeps your blood sugar level on an even keel.
• Eat high-quality foods rich in nutrients – as in the list of superfoods – combined with stimulating and tonic herbs.
• No matter how desperate you are for instant energy, don't fall into the sugar trap. Most people with chronic fatigue at some time reach for the chocolate bar, the sugar bowl or the biscuit tin. They will only make you feel worse.
• Save time and energy in the kitchen: eat lots of raw foods as they mean less work and easier digestion.

3. Sleep

Quality of sleep is more important than quantity. Many people with low-energy levels don't sleep well. They doze during the day and evening and are awake at night-time. This quickly becomes a pattern and regular sleep becomes a thing of the past.

Sleeping pills are not the answer. The quality of sleep they provide is poor and it is common to wake as tired as when you went to bed if you use them.

Get into a regular habit as soon as possible. Set your alarm for seven in the morning, no matter what time you go to bed, and get up when it rings, even if you don't have to. Try not to sleep during the day and avoid late-night stimulants. Drink lime blossom or chamomile tea during the evening instead. If you can't sleep don't just lie there. Get up and do something boring, like the ironing, until you feel tired.

4.   Herbs and spices

There are herbs and spices which are both tonics and stimulants and you should include them in your cooking as well as using some for herbal teas. Parsley, thyme, rosemary, mint, sage, horse-radish, ginger and cinnamon are amongst the best. Grow your own in pots on the kitchen window-sill, or buy fresh ones if you can get them. Dried herbs are almost as good if they are all that is available.

Make tea using two teaspoons of fresh chopped herb or one of dried to a cupful of boiling water. Cover, leave to stand for five minutes, strain, add a little honey if you like, and sip. Use mint, rosemary or half an inch of freshly grated ginger for drinks that will really give you a lift.

5.   Massage

Chronic fatigue causes extreme tension, which in turn wastes much of your valuable energy and leads to more fatigue. Massage removes the tension.

A professional massage is wonderful but there are DIY books and all you need is a willing partner, friend or relative, massage oil and some spare time. As long as your willing pair of hands is not causing any pain it is virtually impossible for massage to do any harm. Start with the big muscles of the back and shoulders; then work in to the buttocks, legs, feet, arms, hands and tummy, using slow rhythmic movements.

Make sure the room is warm, take the phone off the hook and put on some soothing music. Most people will sleep after a massage and wake up refreshed and much more energetic.

6.   All in the mind?

There is no doubt that depression causes loss of energy, but it is equally true that constant fatigue causes depression. It is common for doctors to prescribe anti-depressant drugs and tranquillisers for patients complaining of constant exhaustion. Unfortunately, these drugs interfere with the body's uptake of vital minerals such as iron, zinc and magnesium, which makes the tiredness worse. I am certain that many cases of TAT are caused by these drugs – prescribed for the very symptoms which they are making worse.

In this chicken-and-egg situation, it is far better to help your mind to help your body than it is to rely on drugs. Any of the simple relaxation techniques will help – yoga, meditation or straightforward relaxation exercises – and all can be learned from books or tapes.

7.   Supplements

Taking pills is no substitute for improving your food intake, but the vitamin B group; vitamins A, C and E; and the minerals iron, zinc, magnesium and potassium are essential supplements. Together with Guarana, they should be part of the daily regime to help you cope with chronic fatigue.

The power of Guarana

There is no instant way to extra energy that is safe or provides long-term benefit. Follow this plan for success. Although it might seem hard at first, start right now by making out your shopping list of superfoods, supplements and – especially – Guarana, and you will be amazed at how soon your spirits will soar.

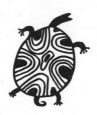

Case history, – ME
Mr, S., age 17, a student

This young man was brought to me in late November by his distraught mother when both of them were just about at their wits' end.

At the end of the previous summer term Mr S. finished the first year of his A-level course. He was taking three subjects, was predicted to get at least two As and a B and was destined for Oxbridge. He was a fit, healthy rugby player and a cross-country runner, heavily involved in many school activities – the choir, amateur dramatics and debating – as well as enjoying his studies. With his extrovert personality, he had a busy social life and a wide circle of friends.

At the end of July this young man went on a family holiday to Greece where he contracted severe food poisoning. He was better within a week and seemed fine, but within two weeks of going back to school his problems began. He started feeling tired, getting headaches and severe pains in various joints and muscles, and eventually he was falling asleep in class. He became too weak to go upstairs to bed, was unable to concentrate on anything for more than a few minutes and generally felt very unwell.

At first his doctor took the matter seriously. After a battery of tests and investigations revealed nothing, it was suggested that he was suffering from stress and anxiety and he was advised to take a course of anti-depressant drugs. Happily his mother refused to allow this, but by now the doctors and the school were convinced that he was suffering from depression.

By the time I saw this unfortunate young fellow he really was depressed – but as a result of his illness, not as the cause of it.. I was convinced that here was a case of ME and referred him to Professor Mowbray at St Mary's Hospital, London, who is one of the few eminent researchers in this field. Blood tests confirmed the presence of antibodies to one of the viruses linked with ME and the professor's diagnosis was unequivocal: He was certain that this patient did have ME.

We instituted a regime of extremely healthy eating, lots of rest and absolutely no pressure on him to perform or 'pull his socks up'. He was taking a range of vitamin and mineral supplements and very slowly but surely he started to improve. After my first visit to the Amazon, I had been so impressed with what I had learned about Guarana that I added four capsules of this remarkable plant together with two cups of Guarana tea each day to his regular regime. Within a week he telephoned me to say how much better and more energetic he was feeling. From this point on his whole recovery accelerated. In fact the major problem was to stop him doing too much too soon, undoing the good work of his gradual recovery.

Having missed most of the winter term, by the time the Christmas holidays were over he returned to school. Although he was still not able to take part in any sporting activities, he completed his A-level course and went happily on to university. There is no doubt in my mind that adding Guarana to this treatment shortened his period of recovery by at least six months and that without it he would not have had success in his A-levels.

Case history – SAD
Miss B., age 27, executive with major PR company

It was five o'clock on a dark cold February afternoon when Miss B. sat in my consulting room, the tears streaming down her face. 'I can't go on like this any longer, so I've decided to hand in my notice', she sobbed. Here was a typical case of Seasonal Affective Disorder, better known as SAD. We've always known about the 'winter blues', but most people believed that it was simply a wish for warmer and sunnier weather. Today SAD is officially recognised as being a genuine medical problem. Up to two million people – 80% of them women – are thought to suffer its consequences in the UK alone.

Miss B. was typical. As the winter progressed she became miserable and depressed for no obvious reason. She had uncontrollable cravings for sweet and starchy foods and each year between November and the spring she gained around one-and-a-half stone, spending the next six months struggling to get it off again. She seemed to need more and more sleep and yet she woke tired every morning. She stopped going out and had no interest in sexual activity, and coping with her job became virtually impossible. Her fiancé broke off their engagement and the only help she had been offered by her doctor was yet another course of anti-depressant drugs. She had already tried these for two consecutive winters with absolutely no benefit.

The cause of SAD is now known to be the hormone melatonin. It is released from the pineal gland in the brain during the night. Thanks to the pioneering research of psychiatrist Dr Alfred Lewy and Dr Richard Wurtman, professor of endocrinology at the Massachusetts Institute of Technology, we now know that light entering the eye affects the pineal gland and inhibits the release of melatonin. During the bright sunny days of spring and summer the amount of this hormone circulating in the body is very low. As the days get shorter it rises, mimicking the patterns of hibernation in animals.

The answer has been found, thanks to science and technology, to be exposure to bright light. Studies have now shown that for many SAD sufferers sitting in front of a simple light box emitting ten thousand lux can make a dramatic difference.

Miss B. acquired a light box and we made a great effort to improve her nutrition. Her diet included more complex carbohydrates, lots of beta-carotene-rich foods, simple proteins and small meals at a maximum of three-hourly intervals. The greatest problem was to tide her over the period during which the treatment would take effect. In her depressive state everything became an insurmountable problem.

Large doses of Guarana – two 500 mg capsules three times a day for one week, then reduced to twice a day for three months, was enough to do the trick. The stimulus of the Guarana gave her the energy to overcome the short-term problem. The light box and the improved nutrition resolved it completely. She kept her job and three years on has not had another bad winter.

Case history – TAT
Mr W., age 56, divorced, redundant machine-tool operator

It is patients like Mr W. that make my blood boil. As a middle-aged, redundant, divorced man living on his own, he is automatically pigeon-holed. After doing the rounds of specialists and having a battery of tests, he was finally brought to me by his sister, who was certain that his problems were caused by his bad eating habits.

He had been divorced and living on his own for just over two years and was then made redundant after nineteen years with the same company. He lived modestly, had some savings and received a handsome redundancy payment from his company, so he had no pressing financial problems. For two or three months he scoured the job market, then realised that at his age he was unlikely to find full-time employment. He got a small part-time job which he enjoyed, but gradually found himself becoming more and more tired and lethargic. He gave up his part-time job, stopped going to the bowls club and spent an ever-increasing amount of time in bed. But no matter how much he slept, it did not seem to make any difference.

He had been tested for anaemia, thyroid problems, cancer, leukaemia and almost every disease known to mankind. At the end of the day the doctors popped him neatly into his pigeon-hole and labelled him as a depressive. He was prescribed anti-depressant drugs and after three months on these felt no more cheerful and even more tired. By now the doctors were suggesting psychiatric treatment and at this point his sister put her foot down.

Yes, Mr W. was typical, but not a typical depressive. He had lost his wife and his job but had coped with these with his normal sense of good humour. The thing which had changed the most in his lifestyle was his diet. He had previously never done more cooking than putting on the kettle, popping down the toaster, or at a push, boiling an egg. His diet now was mainly take-aways, bread and cheese, beans on toast and the occasional fry-up, all washed down with copious amounts of strong tea. While he was still working full-time he was getting a couple of filled rolls in the morning and a good hot meal in the works canteen at lunch-time, but when this stopped his nutritional decline began.

There are many nutritional problems which do not cause obvious deficiency diseases like scurvy, rickets or beri-beri. Whilst our Mr W. was probably getting enough calories and enough protein, his intake of other nutrients was marginal. The result was a gradual decline in some of the essential requirements of the diet. Millions of people limp through life with marginal sub-clinical malnutrition. We do not all get enough of the nutrients that we need, and in any case there is often a considerable difference between the amount of any specific essential substance which is necessary to sustain life and the amount which the body needs for optimum health.

In 1985 a survey in Britain indicated that 35% of all men, and 67% of all women, had an intake of zinc that fell alarmingly short of the 11 mg per day recommended by the World Health Organization. It is almost certainly zinc which is a major part of Mr W.'s problem. A lack of zinc, together with too little iron and magnesium, is the commonest cause of Tired All the Time syndrome. Anti-depressant drugs interfere with the body's absorption of these minerals, leading to greater fatigue and so exacerbating the very condition with which he went to the doctor in the first place. Add to this all the tea, which contains tannins that also interfere with mineral uptake, and you can easily understand his downward spiral.

In this situation the first requirement is to increase the general level of energy. This was done by regular doses of Guarana, 1 g in the morning, 500 mg at midday and 500 mg in the late afternoon. Mineral supplements and a good cookbook for beginners combined with a carefully worked-out eating plan were the long-term solutions. Mr W. is back on the bowling green, once again enjoying his part-time job, and has no sign of the TAT which made his life so miserable for so long. Without the Guarana as the initial therapy, he would not have had the energy to put the other steps into practice.

Case history – exhaustion and loss of sex drive
Mr H., age 31, teacher

As Mr H. walked into my consulting room for the first time, that intuitive alarm bell – which you ignore at your peril – went off in my subconcious. Here was a very sick-looking young man: pale, thin, shuffling, with shoulders bent as if he had the cares of the world heaped upon them. My immediate thoughts were that he must be suffering from some major disease – leukaemia, cancer or one of the neurological illnesses. Whatever it was, I was certain that there was some life-threatening process going on within this poor fellow.

His previous medical history was uneventful, with no operations, accidents or serious illness. He had always been a bit on the slim side but enjoyed his job as a teacher and had always helped out on the sports field as well, coaching football, swimming and a bit of tennis in the summer. During the previous six months he had imperceptibly lost weight and slowed down. He had given up all his sporting activities, but had managed to keep on working, to the exclusion of all other interests. He literally got up, went to work, came home and went to bed. He had spent the previous school holidays moping around the house, reading, watching the TV and getting throroughly depressed as he saw his garden turn into a wilderness.

He was now deeply concerned because he had no interest in sex whatsoever and his great fear was that his wife would misinterpret his lack of sexual activity as an indication that he no longer cared for her. The problem was compounded by the fact that shortly before he became ill the couple had decided that it was time to start a family and that his wife – also a teacher – would then give up work.

Mr H. had undergone virtually every test known to medical science. His doctors had been extremely thorough and left no stone unturned to get to the root of this mystery. Sadly, they had drawn a blank at every turn and here he was, sitting in front of me – his last and desperate hope. Being, as I am, committed to the role of nutrition in health, my first question after the initial consultation was to ask about his diet. He was quick to assure me that his wife was a great believer in healthy eating. In fact, as she was a little overweight and as they were thinking of starting a family she had been dieting seriously for some time. On closer questioning it transpired that Mr H's gradual decline coincided with the start of his wife's slimming regime. He had gallantly offered to follow the same diet to give her moral support.

I asked him to keep an exact record of everything he ate and drank over the following seven days. When he brought his list back it was obvious from just a cursory glance that this was not a healthy diet for an active 31-year-old man. His entire intake was fed into my nutritional analysis computer programme, and the result came out as plain as a pikestaff. The 'diet' that his health-concious wife planned for both of them was severely deficient and did not provide even the basic calorie requirements for either of them.

Mr H.   Nutritional Analysis
PERIOD ANALYSED   – Analysis period: 7-day profile
NUTRIENTS ANALYSED   – Nutrients with UK DRVs
RNI GROUP   – 19–50 years moderate–moderately active
Actual intake figures have been divided by 7

NAME	– Mr H.	HEIGHT	– 165.10 cms
AGE	– 31 yrs	WEIGHT	– 50.85 kgms
SEX	– Male		
OCCUPATION	– Moderate	BMI	– 18.66
LIFESTYLE	– Moderate		

% energy FAT	44.3	% energy Sugar	13.2
% energy MUFA	9.3	% energy PROTEIN	13.6
% energy PUFA	4.0	% energy ALCOHOL	1.1
% energy SFA	15.4	Na/K ratio	1.0
% energy Starch	24.6	Na as Salt in gms	6.0
% energy CHO	40.5		

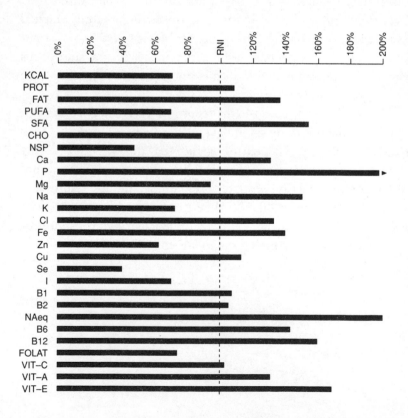

As you will see from his chart, there was an insufficient intake of a number of essential nutrients and an excessive intake of one or two of the undesirables. The vertical line in the middle of the table represents the RNI (the Department of Health's recommended ideal amount) and the horizontal black bars show you the percentage of that ideal amount which is being consumed on average for each of the seven days.

Here is a summary of what I was able to tell him from what the computer told me.

Your diet has been compared with standard Daily Reference Values (DRVs), set by the Department of Health for individuals of different age, sex and activity levels. DRVs have been set at three levels: Reference Nutrient Intakes or maxima, an average and a minimum level of requirement.

A moderate excess of many nutrients is not harmful, but excesses and deficiencies of some nutrients do affect the efficiency with which other nutrients are absorbed and utilised. Amounts exceeding ten times the RNI for vitamins and minerals over a prolonged period may be harmful.

Weight for height
Above or below a range of weights for a given height, the risk of mortality or developing illness increases. The Royal College of Physicians has established standards to achieve optimum health. Your height and weight have been compared with these standards.

The recommendations may not apply if, for example, you are a marathon runner, a weight-lifter, an American footballer or a sumo wrestler. In this case the best assessment, having reached your ideal weight, is whether your weight is steady and whether you are fully fit.

You are considerably underweight for someone of your height. You need to eat more or your health and performance may suffer.

Energy
Energy is measured in kilocalories or kiloJoules and is provided by the metabolism of fats and oils, proteins, carbohydrates (sugars and

starches) and alcohol. Carbohydrate is the most important of the metabolic fuels.

Your requirement for energy has been calculated by applying your personal details to standard equations for calculating metabolic rate.

Energy should be derived in roughly the following proportions:

Energy from protein	8–12% of calories
Energy from fat	33–35% of calories
Energy from saturates	10% of calories
Energy from polyunsaturates	6–10% of calories
Energy from monounsaturates	12% of calories
Energy from carbohydrates	50–60% of calories
Energy from alcohol	No more than 10% of total energy

Your energy intake as reported is low compared with your body weight. You are not eating enough to maintain an acceptable weight for your height.

Protein

Proteins (amino acids) are needed to replace cells and build new tissues. They are components of enzymes and hormones. Any protein in excess of requirements is converted by the body to energy or stored as body fat. There is no evidence that a high protein intake enhances metabolic efficiency or increases muscle bulk.

For most adults in the UK, who have a mixed diet, including vegetarians, there is little reason to be concerned about the amino acid content.

There is evidence that excessive dietary protein may contribute to demineralisation of bone. There is also evidence that excessive dietary protein contributes to renal disease and that animal protein exerts a greater effect than vegetable protein.

Very little known is known about the possible toxic effects of commercially available amino acid supplements and care should be taken if such supplements are used.

Your protein intake is moderately above recommendations but still within prudent limits compared with your weight. The rec-

ommended amount is 0.75 g/kg body weight, which is equivalent
to 38.1 g protein. The protein in your diet came from:

Pizza, cheese and tomato	12.3%
Tea, Indian	9.5%
White bread (average)	7.1%
Pancakes, savoury	6.7%
Prawns, boiled	6.6%
Low fat yogurt, plain	5.6%
Salmon, canned	4.9%

Fat

Fat acts as a carrier for the fat-soluble vitamins and is a concentrated form of energy, providing twice the calories as the same weight
of protein or carbohydrate. All fats – whether butter, margarine,
olive oil or fat on meat – have the same number of calories for a
given weight.

There are many kinds of fats, each with a different chemical
make-up. All fats are a mixture of saturated and unsaturated fatty
acids. The unsaturated fats include the group called polyunsaturat-
ed fats (PUFAs).

Too much fat, and too much saturated fat, can lead to health
problems. A diet high in fat will also contain high levels of cholesterol. There is an increased risk of coronary heart disease from a
diet high in fat, and saturated fat in particular. Cancer of the breast,
colon and prostate are associated with dietary fat.

Dietary fat is a key factor in weight control due to the number
of calories it provides. Obesity is a risk factor in diabetes, hypertension and heart disease.

The proportion of energy derived from fat in your diet is too
high. In the interests of good health and preventing coronary heart
disease you should reduce the amount of fat you eat. These foods
contributed to your total fat intake:

Pancakes, savoury	12.9%
Pizza, cheese and tomato	11.1%
Full fat soft cheese	10.1%

Butter	9.6%
McD donut, cinnamon coating	5.7%
Coconut cake	4.8%

Eat these foods less often or substitute a lower-fat alternative. Make up the calories with starchy carbohydrates like whole-grain bread, pasta and rice.

SFA

Your saturated fat intake is too high. In addition to contributing to total fat, some fats are recognised as risk factors in themselves for coronary heart disease and cancer. Positive health benefits would be achieved by decreasing the amount of non-essential saturated fats in your diet. The saturated fats in your diet came from:

Full fat soft cheese	18.2%
Butter	18.2%
Pizza, cheese and tomato	14.3%

Cholesterol

The cholesterol content of your diet as described is sensible.

Carbohydrates (CHO)

Carbohydrates are an important group of energy foods which include the starches and sugars. The best type are complex carbohydrates; carbohydrates which have not been highly refined or processed – for example, the carbohydrates found in whole-grain bread, pasta, rice, peas and beans, vegetables, fruits and nuts. Refined carbohydrates – for example sweet foods such as sugar, preserves, cakes, biscuits and confectionery – are less useful in the long term.

You are eating too few foods which contain complex carbohydrates for a good balance of energy. Try to eat more whole-grain bread, pasta, cereals, peas and beans, vegetables, fruits and nuts.

Fibre – NSP

Non-starch polysaccharides (NSP) or dietary fibre is a general term applied to a group of carbohydrates found in the walls of plant cells. Animal food products contain none at all. Do not be confused about the various kinds of NSP (whether it is soluble or insoluble, cellulose or non-cellulose); it is all beneficial to health.

Diets high in NSP-rich foods are effective in relieving and preventing constipation. They are also thought to protect against intestinal diseases such as diverticulitis, cancer of the bowel and haemorrhoids. NSP increases faecal weight, which shortens transit time and relieves pressure in the bowels, all of which are beneficial in preventing disorders of the lower bowel.

Research has shown that NSP has a positive effect in reducing blood cholesterol.

It is best to eat foods which are naturally rich in NSP rather than eating bran supplements which contain no other nutrients and which may interfere with the absorption of other nutrients.

NSP-rich foods will fill you up without providing too many calories, useful if you are watching your weight.

The fibre–NSP content of your diet appears to be less than the minimum amount recommended for health. Whole-grain cereals, peas and beans, leafy and root vegetables, fresh and dried fruit and nuts ensure a good supply of fibre as well as providing vitamins, minerals and micronutrients.

Magnesium (Mg)

Magnesium has a role to play in skeletal development and in maintaining electrical impulses in nerve and muscle membranes. Whereas calcium has a stimulating effect on muscle contractility, sodium, potassium and magnesium promote relaxation. Small losses from sweating during exercise can be replaced by vegetables and fruits.

Magnesium is present in many vegetable and animal foods; however, your diet, though including more than the estimated average intake, is below the maximum recommended. Are you sure you are eating a wide variety of foods?

Sodium (Na)

Sodium is used in the maintenance of extracellular fluid for acid-base balance and in sending electrical impulses to muscles and nerves, and it assists in the uptake of nutrients by cells.

About a quarter of the sodium in our diets is naturally present in food. Of the other three-quarters, half comes from the sodium chloride (salt) added to food during processing (meat products, vegetables, soups, breakfast cereals, sauces, pickles, bread, to name a few sources), and a quarter is added during cooking or at the table.

We require so little that most people could get by with just the salt naturally present in unprocessed foods. Salt – whether it is table salt, sea salt, cooking salt or rock salt – is all sodium chloride.

Sodium requirements may increase with unaccustomed hard exercise or exposure to high temperatures, but the body adapts if either type of situation continues.

Your sodium intake is marginally higher than the recommended upper limits. If you suffer from high blood-pressure or there is a history of hypertension or strokes in your family, you should cut down on the salt. The sodium in your diet came from these foods:

Pizza, cheese and tomato	19.7%
Prawns, boiled	11.5%
White bread (average)	11.0%
McD donut, cinnamon coating	4.8%
Hummus (chick pea spread)	4.5%

Potassium (K)

Potassium, like sodium, plays an important part in the acid-base balance of the blood and tissues. Research has shown that potassium minimises the effect of sodium and has a beneficial effect on blood-pressure. Sweating does not significantly deplete body potassium.

Your intake of potassium is lower than the recommended level. Some potassium-rich foods are potatoes, fish, pork, dried fruits, cauliflower, rhubarb, beef, chicken, breakfast cereals, leeks, spinach, sardines, lamb, sweet potatoes, natural yogurt, bananas, fresh fruits, sweetcorn, dried peas and beans and avocados.

Zinc (Zn)

Zinc is an essential component of many enzymes involved in the metabolism of protein, carbohydrate, fats and energy. A feature of deficiency is retarded growth. It is essential to life, but required in very small amounts.

Your intake of zinc is below the average recommended amount. Good sources of zinc are beef, lamb, kidney, liver, breakfast cereals, pork, prawns, sardines, plaice, chicken, Emmenthal and Cheddar cheese, lentils, pumpkin seeds and beans. White bread, fat and sugar are poor sources.

Selenium (Se)

Selenium is part of an enzyme system which acts as an anti-oxidant. There is insufficient evidence to suggest smoking or oral contraceptives increase the requirement for selenium. Neither is there convincing evidence to date that high intakes protect against cancer or cardiovascular disease.

The lower reference intake has been set to maintain tissue saturation.

Your diet as analysed falls below the minimum recommendation for this mineral. Good sources are cereals (especially whole-grain products), meat, fish and eggs. There is very little information available on the amount of selenium in many foods.

Folate

Folate is essential for the formation of red blood cells, growth and cell division. Deficiency leads to anaemia and therefore could have an effect on physical performance. Folic acid is quickly destroyed during cooking.

Your intake of folate is below maximum recommended amounts. Most meat and dairy products contain small amounts. Offal and raw green leafy vegetables are especially rich. Avocados, bananas and oranges are a good source but other fruits have only small amounts.

Vitamin C

Vitamin C is an anti-oxidant. It is required for the normal function of connective tissue, to prevent scurvy and to aid wound healing. Trauma and stress increase the need for it. Drugs, for example aspirin, interfere with its function.

Vitamin C enhances the absorption of iron from vegetables and inhibits nitrosamine formation (a protective function against gastric cancer). Vitamin C may be beneficial to athletes with marginal sports anaemia.

Vitamin C is readily lost from plant foods during storage, on bruising and when cut and exposed to air (salads in salad bars will lose vitamin C). Prolonged boiling in large quantities of water, followed by keeping food hot, can result in the total loss of this vitamin.

Megadoses of this vitamin do not appear to be absorbed and may cause diarrhoea, or may cause the production of kidney stones.

Smokers have an increased turnover of vitamin C and their intake should be *double the maximum requirement.*

Your intake of vitamin C is below the maximum recommendation. Good sources are citrus fruits, blackcurrants, melons, berries of all kinds, raw vegetables, broccoli, brussel sprouts, spring greens, potatoes, spinach, cauliflower, leeks and sweet potatoes.

Vitamin D (calciferols)

Vitamin D is found in very few foods. The major source of this vitamin is the action of sunlight on the skin, which is usually sufficient unless you are confined to the house.

Vitamin D is a precursor of the vitamin which controls the proportion of dietary calcium absorbed and excreted, and it has a direct effect on bones.

The Vitamin D content of your diet is below the recommended amount. Food sources of vitamin D are oily fish (herring, kippers, mackerel, salmon, sardines), liver, eggs and fortified margarines.

I asked Mr H. to come and see me with his wife and gave them both a good talking to about the evils of low calorie diets. Although Mrs H. was a little overweight, the amount of calories in their daily food was nowhere near enough for her either. I pointed out that it was probably fortunate that she had not conceived as the low level of folic acid in their food could cause birth defects. In any case her calorie intake certainly would not have supported a healthy pregnancy either for herself or for a growing foetus.

They were both highly relieved when they understood that the most likely cause of all Mr H.'s problems was basic malnutrition. I immediately advised a course of vitamin and mineral supplements and a dramatic improvement in diet. To overcome the extreme exhaustion which had affected him for so long, I prescribed a three-month course of Guarana. The first essential was to provide Mr H. with an energy boost which would make him better able to cope with his daily life and willing to take more trouble over his nutrition. Within hours of the first dose of Guarana he phoned to say that he was feeling noticeably brighter and within a week of Guarana treatment, vitamins, minerals, better food and more of it, he was cheerful and optimistic.

Within three months this man who had shuffled his way into my room on his first appointment was a stone and a half heavier, looked ten years younger and was bounding with energy. Mrs H. was two months pregnant and blooming, as is the garden, and the school football team are delighted to have their coach back.

The energy-giving properties of Guarana are not just a myth of the Amazon Indians. No pills or potions would have compensated for this patient's poor food consumption, but the Guarana gave him the initial burst of energy that enabled him to cope with his difficulties.

Guarana as an anti-diarrhoeal treatment

As we have seen already at the beginning of this chapter, the rainforest Indians prize Guarana as a specific remedy for diarrhoea. Since I first became aware of this amazing plant medicine I have never travelled without it: from the rainforests of Brazil where I shared the communal cooking pots of the local inhabitants to the vast reaches of the Amazon river living on fish straight out of the water. In the desert plains of the Kalahari in Africa and the hinterlands of the Australian outback in the far north of Queensland, and even in the less hygienic parts of southern Europe, I always take two capsules of Guarana every morning. I have watched in amazement as travelling companions go down like flies with the dreaded 'traveller's tum' whilst I've never had a problem.

Never, that is, except in a posh hotel in São Paulo at the end of one of my visits to the Amazon rainforest. After a few days in a big city in a five-star hotel I stopped taking my daily dose of Guarana. Two days later I ate a hamburger in the hotel restaurant and spent the next forty-eight hours in the loo.

The exceptionally high tannin content of Guarana combined with the fatty saponins ensures a slow gradual release of the mild and protective tannins into the gut, offering round-the-clock protection against invading organisms. I am certain that the rainforest Indians are right. If you are off on your travels, you can gain added protection for your digestive tract from a regular daily dose of Guarana.

6 Why should we take Guarana seriously?

Before examining the specific health benefits of a single plant medicine such as Guarana, it is vital to understand the immeasurable importance of this plant as an example of the role of plant medicines. We must take the story of Guarana seriously. For a number of ecological, economical, environmental and, above all, humanitarian reasons, this story serves to illustrate the loss there will be on a global scale if the world at large fails to take potentially valuable plants seriously.

As far back as 1986 scientists had become alarmed by the destruction of the rainforests. At that time Professor Edward Wilson of Harvard University in the USA calculated that around 36,000 squares miles of rainforest were falling to the chainsaw every year – an area equivalent to the size of Switzerland and Holland put together. There were concerns about the impact on weather and the indigenous tribes. Thousands of plant species had already been destroyed, an irreversible loss to the biodiversity of our planet and an incalculable loss in terms of undiscovered medicines that might have been used to alleviate human suffering.

According to the journal of the Herb Research Foundation in America published in 1987, anxiety over the extinction of many plant species had even been raised in the American Congress. In September 1986 the House of Representatives legislated for the US Agency for International Development to earmark a budget of $10 million to be used for the preservation of biodiversity. Professor Wilson commented:

> While scientists and environmentalists may hail such a move, the amount budgeted is much too small to make an effective impact on the situation, not to mention the possibility of being too late. The time has come to link ecology to economic and human development ... what is happening to the rain forests of Madagascar and Brazil will affect us all.

In 1989 the Assembly of the World Health Organization adopted a resolution in support of traditional medicine and drew attention to herbal medicines as being of great importance to the health of individuals and communities. How tragic it is that governments and drug regulatory authorities in the UK, most of the rest of Europe and the USA continue to turn a convenient blind eye. The WHO estimates that 80% of the world's population depends mainly on local traditional medicines for health care. Despite the apparent official dismissal of the value of phytotherapy and seemingly tireless efforts by governments to restrict its availability, it remains true that 25% of all prescriptions are for medicines containing plant extracts.

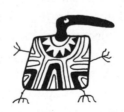

The advent of sulphonamides and antibiotics and the 'magic bullets' approach to drug research have slowly but surely pushed the importance of plant medicines into the shade. Happily the general public, disillusioned with side-effects, adverse reactions and a growing number of highly publicised drug disasters, has developed a healthy scepticism about the products of the pharmaceutical industry. With a dramatic swing of the pendulum people are turning to alternative therapies in general and most specifically to self-medication with herbal remedies. But this is only a fraction of the story. Within the bounds of orthodox scientific medicine, drugs derived directly from plants – even those now synthesised by biotechnology – are of unquestionably major importance in the physician's armoury. It is interesting to speculate how many of the doctors writing prescriptions, the majority of whom would question the value of 'herbal medicines', are aware of the origins of the highly potent drugs they are prescribing.

According to Professor Norman Farnsworth:

No one would seriously challenge the fact that man is still largely dependent on plants in treating his ailments. According to an estimate of the WHO, approximately 88% of people in developing countries rely chiefly on traditional medicines (mostly plant extracts) for their primary health care needs. In the People's Republic of China, with a population of more than one billion, the main type of drug therapy is still in the form of plant extracts. This high degree of dependence, based on trial and error over many generations, is surely a demonstration of efficacy: these plants and/or their extracts would not have remained in use unless they provided some relief from symptoms. Even in the United States, where synthetics dominate the drug market scene, plant products still represent an important source of prescription drugs. Approximately one fourth of all prescriptions dispensed from community pharmacies in the United States contain one or more ingredients derived from the higher plants which in 1980 was valued at $8.112 billion.
(*Perspectives in Biology and Medicine*, 32, 2, Winter 1989)

Farnsworth has made a computerised analysis of plant-derived medicines which reveals that there are 121 prescription drugs in common use which owe their origins to plants. Only about forty of these are available in the USA, owing to FDA regulations. Of the ninety-five species of plant which yield the 121 medicines, thirty-nine have their homes in tropical rainforests and are responsible for the production of forty-seven prescription medicines.

These are not 'herbal remedies' shrouded in folklore and mystic rites, nor are they left-overs from the flower power 1960s. They are major drugs used at the cutting edge of modern scientific medicine – drugs which physicians and patients alike have good cause to be thankful for.

- **Atropine** *(Atropa belladonna)* Used for dilating the pupils prior to examination or surgery, for the treatment of slow heartbeat, in Parkinson's disease, asthma and severe diarrhoea, and issued to military personnel during the Gulf War as an antidote to nerve gas.
- **Cocaine** *(Erythroxylum coca)* A local anaesthetic.
- **Vinblastine** and **vincristine** *(Catharanthus roseus,* the Madagascan rosy periwinkle) used for the treatment of Hodgkin's disease and childhood leukaemias.
- **Quinine** and **quinidine** *(Cinchona ledgeriana)* Vital anti-malarial; and its derivative, used to treat most types of irregular heartbeats.
- **Pilocarpine** *(Pilocarpus jaborandai)* used for the treatment of glaucoma.
- **L-dopa** *(Mucuna deeringiaa)* Has revolutionised the treatment of Parkinson's disease.
- **Diosgenin** *(Dioscorea mexicana)* Produced from the Mexican yam and used to synthesise corticosteroids, sex hormones and oral contraceptives.
- **Ouabain** *(Strophanthus gratus)* Like digitalis, this is a cardiac gly-coside used for acute heart failure.
- **Papain and Chymopapain** *(Carica papava)* Used in the treatment of ulcers, burns and wounds, and in disc surgery.
- **d-Tubocurarine** *(Strychnos* and *Chondodendron,* the active ingredient in curare from the Amazon and a powerful muscle relaxant) Synthesised and used in almost every 'pre-med' to avoid deep anaesthesia.
- **Reserpine** *(Rauwolfia serpentina)* One of the earliest effective blood-pressure lowering drugs.
- **Scopolameine** *(Hyoscyamus niger,* also known as hyacine)

Similar to atropine, used as a pre-med before surgery, for motion sickness and in Parkinson's disease.

- **Physostigmine** (*Physostigma venenosum*) Used to constrict the pupil of the eye and reduce pressure inside the eyeball in the treatment of glaucoma.

These major drugs are derived from plants which grow only in the tropical forests. But the question that has to be asked is this. Statistically it is much more likely that tropical rainforest plants will have some beneficial medical effect than that temperate plants will. Some three thousand plants growing in the Brazilian rainforest alone may have healing properties. So why are we not seeing new drugs derived from these plants appearing, month in and month out?

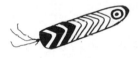

The answer is two-fold. It is partly due to attitude and partly due to money.

The attitudes in question are those of both the pharmaceutical companies and the drug-regulating authorities, combined with the entrenched attitudes of many scientists. As we head towards the millenium, the ecologists, environmentalists, meterorologists and above all millions of concerned earth dwellers look on in seemingly helpless horror as the rainforests disappear. The indigenous inhabitants are exploited, murdered or driven out. Cattle barons, mineral miners and corrupt politicians move in. And with the best will in the world governments whose countries are in the most dire financial crisis seem unable, unwilling or both, to halt the inevitable. The total destruction of the rainforests seems likely by the early twenty-first century.

Time is running out and the renewable resources are rapidly becoming non-renewable. The development of important drugs from the rainforest flora, and the potentially massive financial rewards that they could bring, may be the only route to salvation and conservation for the rainforests. Action must be taken, and taken urgently, to launch massive research campaigns and to ensure just financial rewards if there is to be any chance of success.

The peoples who inhabit the forest must benefit, the countries where the forests grow must benefit, naturally the drug companies must benefit. Above all, mankind will benefit – as it has already through the bounty of naturally occurring plant medicines.

Some of the most powerful plant chemicals are the alkaloids, and their value is most dramatically indicated in the derivatives of the Madagascan periwinkle, vinblastine and vincristine, now used throughout the world in the treatment of childhood leukaemias and Hodgkin's disease. These two drugs alone represent a $100 million a year industry and you would expect that they would generate a healthy return for Madagascar. In fact Madagascar has gained nothing from these drugs from which we benefit so widely in the developed world. It is a major priority to see that the countries of origin of the plants which yield our future drugs get a fair share of the rewards.

But it is not just money that they need. A 1991 workshop sponsored by the US Agency for International Development, the National Science Foundation and the National Institutes of Health brought together interested parties from around the world to explore drug development, biological diversity and economic growth. One of the problems evident from the discussions was the enormous length of time that elapsed between the identification of a plant-derived potential medicine and its availability as a prescription drug – something between ten and fifteen years. Many of the countries where the rich harvest of plants grow are in such dire financial straits that they are unlikely to have either the means or the incentive to institute and maintain conservation programmes, if they have to wait so long for any financial return.

Drug companies could possibly help with technology transfer, developing an infrastructure to identify, collect and study botanical specimens. They could make drugs available for the treatment of local tropical diseases; they could help to finance processing companies so that plant materials could be reduced to refined extracts at source. This would result in job-creation schemes and vitally needed hard currency revenue.

The American National Cancer Institute, which has restarted its massive programme of collecting and testing plant products in the search for anti-cancer and anti-HIV agents, is now adding six thousand new samples a year to its research database. The NCI plans to ensure that any marketable drug developed as a result of its own samples, whether by itself or by an outside pharmaceutical company, will bring adequate compensation to the host country of the plant.

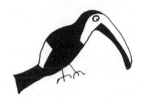

Even our leading medical journals are taking up the cudgels on behalf of ethnic plant medicines. The *British Medical Journal* in its 8 January 1994 edition carried this story from Jan Rocha, Brazil correspondent of *The Guardian*:

> Brazilian scientists are worried about the destruction of the Amazon rainforest and the smuggling out of plants by foreign researchers.
>
> At the 'earth summit' in Rio de Janeiro last year Brazil's former environment secretary, Jose Lutzenberger, warned, 'The pharmaceutical companies have hundreds of researchers combing forests throughout the world, talking to Indians to discover plants with medicinal qualities, and sending back botanical material. Then we shall have to pay royalties to use the medicines developed from them.'
>
> At the first international symposium on the chemistry of the Amazon, held in Brazil last month, his concerns were reinforced by the chairman, Dr Peter Rudolf Seidl. He gave an

example of the practice that drugs were being developed by the National Institutes of Health in the US that included parts of Amazonian plants found by researchers from New York Botanical Gardens.

'We don't want to stop researchers coming here but we do want their research shared with Brazil, to be in partnership with our institutions.' Dr Siedl said that local communities should be paid for their knowledge and natural resources and that researchers should ensure that their lifestyle was not disturbed. 'These lifestyles are essential to the preservation of the segment of the rainforest in which the communities live,' he said.

The symposium published a statement warning that, in spite of recommendations from the earth summit and the efforts of government and non-government organisations, Amazonian biodiversity was being destroyed faster than ever. The statement calls for 'myths about Amazonian biodiversity to be removed so that its economic significance or market value can be objectively assessed. Conditions for negotiating the transfer of knowledge presently held by local populations for the extraction of raw materials and the introduction of processes that add value to the products of the region should be established.'

The scientists who were at the symposium want investigations on biodiversity to be carried out in the Amazon region. Brazil has several research institutes, such as the National Amazon Research Institute and the Emilio Goeldi Museum; they all suffer from lack of funding and staff owing to constant changes in government policy.

The minister for the environment and the Amazon, Rubens Ricupero, said: 'Under the biodiversity convention approved at the earth summit, which comes into effect this month, every discovery made from a natural product belonging to one country must include that country in its benefits.'

If the Lewises, running a small friendly business from the sea-side town of Brighton in England, can achieve these goals with Guarana, why is it not happening throughout the world? With no support from outside government agencies, without the vast financial resources of the major pharmaceutical companies, but solely through their own ethical approach to business, they are resolute in their determination to see that local rainforest inhabitants have a major incentive to protect their environment. They achieve this by dealing with local gatherers and processors of the plant and seeing that they get fair rewards for their labours. Maintaining the integrity of the forest is the key to their livelihood and survival.

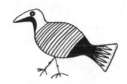

The real stumbling block, which stands in the way of major new drug development from plants and a worldwide incentive to translate conservation from talk into action, is an attitude problem. It is the attitude of the majority of western scientists to what they imagine to be the myth and magic of herbal medicines. Varro E. Tyler, professor of pharmacognosy at Purdue University, Indiania, presented a fascinating paper at the Tropical Forest Medical Resources and the Conservation of Biodiversity Symposium held in January 1992 at the Institute of Economic Botany, The Rockefeller University, New York City. He opened his paper with this wonderful story:

> Some time in prehistory, in the part of the world that is now the country of Peru, a raging storm felled a giant tree which came to rest in a pool of stagnant water. It lay there for some time, the water leaching the various constituents – tannins, glycosides, sugars, and alkaloids – from the bark of the tree. Eventually, a native passed that way. He was extremely ill, burning with the fever which Hippocrates

called intermittent, which during the Middle Ages was
known as the ague, and which we today call malaria. His
fever had caused intense thirst, and he drank copiously from
the pond. Shortly thereafter a miracle occurred, and his
fever vanished. The disease that proved fatal to such well-
known victims as Alexander the Great had undergone
remission.

Whether the native drank repeatedly from the pool as the
fever recurred and how it was that he associated his cure
with the bark of the immense tree lying in the water, we do
not know. We do not really know if this imagined scenario
approaches the truth relative to the discovery of the utility
of cinchona bark in treating malaria. But it is possible,
because at some time, some place, something like this had to
happen so human beings could wrest the secret of the fever
bark tree and use it to cure human ailments.

However it was that early humans identified the healing plants,
whether by accident, whether by trial and error, or whether by
some divine intervention, is unimportant. The plain truth is that
five thousand years ago the Chinese had written records of herbal
medicines. Over three thousand years ago the Ebers Papyrus contained specific prescriptions for medicines – such as roasted and
ground-up paste of ox liver for night blindness, which would have
worked because of its vitamin A content. More than 1,900 years
ago *De Materia Medica*, Dioscorides' landmark book, listed six
hundred medicinal plants, the majority of which are still used by
modern herbalists and some of which are used in conventional
drugs. But even more important than the writings of these early
academics is the vast store-house of knowledge passed on by word
of mouth from family to family, from tribe to tribe, from generation to generation.

   If we destroy the forests we destroy their peoples and we not only
lose plants of immense potential to alleviate human suffering; we
also lose the knowledge which could point us in the right direction.
According to Dr Ryan Huxtable from the University of Arizona,

10% of plants tested at random show some degree of anti-cancer activity. Random testing for anti-HIV activity results in 6% of positive testing. But if the testing is confined to plants that are known to be used traditionally by local inhabitants for specific properties, then the success rate can be double or more: 20% for cancer, 29% for anti-parasitic drugs, and 25% of plants used in viral illness for anti-HIV activity.

Huxtable is eloquent in his plea for plant and animal preservation, quoting as examples the Madagascar periwinkle, the Pacific yew, leeches and, especially, the *Ginkgo biloba*. This last, the oldest surviving tree, was only saved from extinction by early temple plantings. The Ginkgo is used throughout China and Europe – it is the basis of one of the medicines currently most prescribed in Germany – and it has immense value in the treatment of confusion and memory loss in the elderly and in Alzheimer's disease. What is more, it has the potential for treating one of the major neurosurgery problems, post-operative swelling of the brain tissue.

It is only by chance that the value of some plants was revealed before their extinction. As Huxtable says:

> For every success there must have been 100 failures of which we are unaware. We can only speculate as to what has been irretrievably lost ... it is a sad fact of human psychology that we miss what we have had but give little consideration to what we could have had.

The common attitude of the medical and pharmaceutical researcher is to dismiss all folk medicines as hocus pocus. What we need is the combined input of the ethnobotanist, the anthropologist, the botanist, the pharmacologist, the chemist and the medicine men from the university of the forest as well as from the university medical school. Dr Elaine Elisabetsky of the Universidad Federal do Paro in Brazil summed up the situation succinctly: 'A traditional remedy is not a natural product, it's a product of human knowledge. Using this knowledge to search for active compounds could reduce costs as well as time, compared with random mass screening.'

That brings us full circle. In the past tribal medicine men have shared many of their secrets, and generations of their accumulated wisdom, with western scientists without thought of reward. They have frequently been exploited and it is now time to see that this does not happen again. It costs around $200 million to develop a new drug from its inception to its prescription by your doctor, and the drug companies need to recoup this investment. As we have seen with the Madagascan periwinkle, when you end up with a $100 million-a-year business it does not take so very long. But drug companies need formulae which they can patent, chemicals with which they can play molecular roulette to make their product unique and uncopiable – in short to make sure that their new drug has a monopoly in the field.

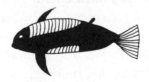

Why invest millions in studying the feverfew plant when anyone can grow it in their own garden and treat their own migraine? Why spend years working on mint or ginger when the requirements of governments mean you have to prove safety and efficacy at vast cost, while anybody can buy them in the corner store and turn them into tea to treat indigestion or morning sickness in pregnancy?

Professor Huxtable tells us why, and in no uncertain terms, in his definitive review article 'The Pharmacology of Extinction', (*Journal of Ethnopharmacology*, 37, 1992, Elsevier Ireland). He gives us examples of species believed to be inconsequential and useless until science found otherwise and of those which, but for the grace of some accidental intervention, we would never have known about or been able to benefit from.

Ginkgo biloba, commonly known as the maidenhair tree – at first glance its leaves have a resemblance to the maidenhair fern – is a survivor from 190 million years ago. As previously mentioned, the Ginkgo became extinct as a forest tree in China many centuries ago and survived only because it had been planted at temple entrances for ornamental purposes. It was first grown in Europe in the botanic gardens in Utrecht in Holland in the early 1700s, and was introduced to the southern states of the USA in the early nineteenth century. This extraordinary survivor from prehistory is extremely tough and grows in conditions that would be impossible for most other trees. Atmospheric pollution, exhaust fumes and extremes of temperature do little to affect its growth.

Extracts from *Ginkgo biloba* have been used in Chinese herbal medicine for centuries to lower blood-pressure, and modern studies of its pharmacology have revealed an extraordinary range of potential value to mankind. This unique material has the potential to control irregular heart beats, prevent spasm of the airways and possibly to be valuable in the treatment of asthma, to be useful in the prevention of graft rejection and in the treatment of shock and stroke; there is even the possibility of its use in transplant patients as a safer form of immunosuppressant. Huxtable concludes, 'All in all this adventitious survivor from the age of the dinosaurs has interesting, intriguing and useful pharmacological activities, having relevance to a range of clinical problems'.

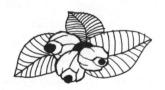

And there is Pacific yew. Here we see a prime example of human stupidity and arrogance, for it has been assumed that this tree is no more than a nuisance and has absolutely no value. A native of the Pacific north-west that takes up to two hundred years to reach a mere forty feet, it has been grubbed out and destroyed to make room for bigger and bigger plantations of quick-growing conifers as cash crops. The result is that 90% of the Pacific yews in North America have vanished and it is now an endangered species.

In 1971 a chemical called taxol was found in Pacific yew. Whilst this terpenoid has been found in other varieties, it is only present in them in very small amounts. Researchers discovered that taxol is a valuable drug in the treatment of ovarian cancer and can have a 40% success rate in halting this disease – which kills twelve thousand women a year in the United States alone. Taxol is now being used in the treatment of breast cancer as well, and the latest reports indicate a 50% success rate.

But now we face a problem. According to the American National Cancer Institute, we have to resolve 'the ultimate conflict between medicine and the environment.' Huxtable tells us:

> available stands of yew are now insufficient even to begin to meet the demand for this drug. Increased harvesting is opposed by those concerned with maintaining a sufficient population of the species, however one root of problem is the earlier unconsidered destruction of much of the population of the Pacific yew.

What an irony, that Bristol-Myers Squibb Pharmaceuticals have just released taxol as a licensed product for the treatment of ovarian cancer where other standard therapies have failed.

Huxtable even manages to point the finger of accusation at religion. In Chapter 1 Mark Plotkin's observation that every time a medicine man dies it is like burning down a library is quoted. Huxtable reinforces this sad thought in relation to the Aztecs and other Meso-American cultures. These peoples made full use of the plants available to them and had an extraordinary knowledge of their local ethnobotany. Though the plants which they used have not vanished from our planet, the knowledge which they had accumulated over centuries and passed down from generation to generation has. It was eradicated and destroyed by the Spanish Conquistadores as they introduced the concept of Christianity to southern America – anyone who has seen the film *The Mission* will have grasped the enormity of the cultural damage done in the name of Christianity. If you missed the film, get the video, it is a thought-provoking and horrendous story.

A tiny but highly important proportion of the plants used by the Aztecs were powerful hallucinogens, used by the Indians in religious ceremonies. Not until 1939 was part of the mystery unravelled. For centuries it was thought that the Ololiuqui – the Aztec name for a type of seed used in divination ceremonies – was a member of the *Solanaceae* family. But in 1939, growing in an Indian garden in Mexico, was found the true plant of the Ololiuqui, *Rivea corymbosa*, a member of the *Convolvulaceae* and a true morning glory. The Aztec world had been destroyed for four hundred years and its destroyer, the Spanish empire, had long since vanished, yet the plant survived.

These hallucinogens are more than a relic of the flower power era and have important applications in modern medicine.

Professor Huxtable illustrates the need for worldwide concern at the loss of even what appears to be the least significant species on our planet. It would be hard to find better words than his to summarise the critical situation which is apparent to the dedicated few; worrying to the growing body of informed general public; yet ignored by governments, legislators and multi-national companies.

Each of the examples discussed is a success story in the history of ethnopharmacology. For every success, however, there must have been a hundred failures of which we are unaware. We can only speculate as to what has been irretrievably lost with the vast and accelerating number of man-induced extinctions of plants, insects, animals and birds. It is a sad fact of human psychology that we miss what we have had but give little consideration to what we could have had.

Natural products are an irreplaceable source of novel compounds. What modern chemist would think of synthesizing compounds such as taxol, vincristine or dolastatin 10 without the stimulus of finding it in nature or a preliminary indication that it will be useful?

The Canadian writer, Robertston Davies (1988) defines a Philistine as 'someone who is content to live in a wholly unexplored world'. 'What use is it?' the Philistine asks when he hears that the construction of a dam is threatening the survival of the snail darter, a small fish. However, as Dryden remarks, 'Everything in the world is good for something'. One cannot predict which unconsidered species may suddenly spring to pharmacological prominence. Use and uselessness are constructs of the mind, an artificial duality having no place in nature. The inability to see a use for an unconsidered and threatened species is a failure of imagination – the type of failure that saw the Atlantic as a vast and stormy waste, bounding and limiting Europe rather than as a great highway to the undiscovered variety of the New World.

Progress in pharmacology and neuroscience continues to depend on the study of novel natural products. For such progress to continue, the ethnobotanical knowledge of vanishing cultures must be recorded and the accelerating rate of man-induced extinction of plant species slowed.

Man is a poor organic chemist compared to nature and nature will continue to inspire our synthetic efforts. We can only wonder at what have been lost forever with the heedless and accelerating extermination of plant species over the last few decades.

As we have seen in this chapter, there are environmental, social, economic and medical reasons for protecting threatened areas of our world. We can no longer afford to consider short-term financial gain in place of long-term global strategy. We must not ignore what seem to be insignificant plants or creatures inhabiting our planet. We cannot continue to tamper with ecosystems which have evolved through aeons of time. We must not displace people from their homelands and eradicate their cultures, and above all we dare not ignore the knowledge of the shamans and the medicine men. As the population of this globe increases and with it the social deprivation of millions upon millions of its inhabitants, as science pushes the survival of humans far beyond three score years and ten, we will need all the help we can get from nature.

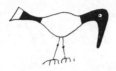

There are battles to be fought and won. Battles against cancer, AIDS and Alzheimer's disease. Battles against malnutrition. Even battles against everyday minor ailments. What is the purpose of increasing the quantity of life if we cannot maintain its quality? Nothing must be ignored in our search for the ultimate goal – the goal of good health. Consider the story of the sea hare. These shell-less molluscs have no monetary value and are apparently of no use to mankind, so who would care if they vanished from the face of the earth? Their one interesting function is that they produce a chemical which causes blisters if you handle them. But now we know that this defensive secretion contains at least nine chemicals which could have anti-cancer activity every bit as powerful as the vincristine extracted from the Madagascan rosy periwinkle.

The rainforests of Brazil host the world's biggest collection of plants with the potential for medical use. What you have read in this chapter should make you realise that it is not possible to hazard even the wildest guess at the benefits to mankind which have already gone up in smoke as the forests burn. It is not possible to estimate the potential for good that still lies waiting for us on the forest floor; in the bark of the trees, in the fruits, nuts, seeds, flowers and roots which proliferate with such abundance in nature's pharmacy.

Thanks to the rainforest Indians, much knowledge survives. We are only now beginning the journey of pharmacological exploration which will lead us to a greater understanding of the benefits of plants such as Guarana.

7 Guarana – The Evidence

Solely as a result of my own personal experiences, I have become increasingly interested in Guarana as a very useful and beneficial natural plant product. Before my first visit to the Brazilian rainforest I already had some knowledge of the traditional Indian uses for this medicine, particularly as an aid to coping with extremes of heat and as an effective mood enhancer. How accurate the knowledge of the Maués-Saterés Indians turned out to be.

Two of the things I dislike most in life are heat and humidity, so imagine my immense discomfort, having boarded a plane at London's Heathrow on a frosty October night, on stepping out at Manaus airport in the heart of the Amazonian rainforest. It was over 100° with 94% humidity. In seconds I was drenched in sweat and that's pretty much how I stayed for the next two weeks: uncomfortable, irritable, bad-tempered and lethargic. That's how I was until the Guarana started to take effect. Within a couple of days of taking it I was the epitome of sweetness and light, bounding with energy and, although I was by far the oldest member of our group, there were younger and fitter fellow travellers struggling to keep up with me.

Can Guarana increase energy and reduce stress?

Was it all in the mind? Was it just an example of a placebo effect? I don't think so, nor do the hundreds of people whom I have advised to take Guarana during the past four years. Three quite simple studies demonstrate the potential of this plant. The first two were carried out at the State Hospital of Copenhagen by Bo Netterstrom. He was aware that the Danes had a growing interest in natural medicines, especially those which seemed to offer a combination of mental and physical stimulation. He singled out Guarana because of its content of the chemical guaranine – a tetramethylxanthine – and its reputation for promoting energy, improving overall vitality and countering stress. He also chose it because of its apparent lack of side-effects.

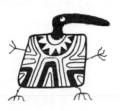

Netterstrom reports that as well as guaranine, present in the natural product in concentrations of between 3 and 5%, Guarana was also alleged to contain a number of other substances which were mostly saponins – which is not unexpected as the plant is a member of the soapwood family or *Sapindaceae* – salts, tannin as tannic acid and small amounts of theobromine and theophylline. In analyses sodium was the most predominant of the salts. In 1989 Netterstrom set up a small double-blind study using a placebo and Guarana, with the object of observing the subjective effects of the product and identifying any side-effects produced by normal use.

Six volunteers who all worked at the Rigshospitalet (the National Hospital, Copenhagen) and who considered themselves to be generally in good health were asked to take part in this study. Five of them were women and one a man, and their ages ranged from 35 to 48 years old.

The study began at the end of October 1989 and ran for eight weeks. Before commencement each of the volunteers had his or her blood-pressure recorded and a blood analysis was undertaken to examine levels of haemoglobin, sedimentation, alkaline phosphatase, creatinine, IgE, cholesterol, fibrinogen, platelets, alanine, aminotransferase (ALT) and glycosylated haemoglobin (Hb_1Ac).

The volunteers were randomly divided into two groups by drawing lots, one being the Guarana group and the other the placebo group. The Guarana group – four participants – were given two 500 mg capsules of Guarana on an empty stomach in the morning and again in the evening each day. The other group – two participants – were given placebo capsules. At the end of four weeks the two participants from the placebo group and the four from the Guarana group had their blood sampled again and all participants in each group had their medication reversed. The placebo group were now receiving Guarana and the Guarana group were now being given a placebo for a further four weeks. At the end of each four-week period all the participants were questioned about their subjective feelings during the previous four weeks and asked to report on any physiological changes or side-effects.

Although this was a very simple small-scale observational study and the sample is not large enough to lead to any statistical conclusions, the results were sufficiently interesting to encourage Netterstrom to do a follow-up study over a longer period of time. In this experiment one of the volunteers discontinued the trial after two weeks due to a slight tendency to oedema (fluid retention), but the others all completed the full eight weeks.

Four out of the remaining five participants showed a slight weight loss during their time on Guarana, the maximum for any one subject being 2 kg in four weeks. Three out of the five reported that they had a subjective feeling of having more energy and being less tired during their period on Guarana but they did not notice the same effect whilst on the placebo. The fifth subject reported no obvious changes. None of the subjects observed any changes in his or her perception of stress but none of the volunteers in the study considered him or herself to be a particularly stressed individual.

Of all the blood tests performed during the study the only one that showed any change was the level of fibrinogen. During the periods on Guarana all the patients registered a drop in the fibrinogen content of their blood. This reduction did not occur during the placebo period.

Raised levels of fibrinogen are associated with stress and are considered to be a specific risk factor for heart disease. The links between heart disease and stress are clearly established and any non-toxic medication which helps to reduce fibrinogen levels could have an important role to play in reducing the current epidemic of premature deaths from heart disease.

Netterstrom concluded that his double-blind test covering an eight-week period established that Guarana had a positive effect relative to the participants' subjective feelings of being more energetic. The test also showed a slight but measurable weight loss in some of the participants and a drop in fibrinogen levels was also found. Netterstrom thought these findings were encouraging enough to warrant further studies, preferably over a much longer period of time, to establish any additional benefits and to isolate any side-effects – apart from the one case of fluid retention, which he felt could be related to the sodium content of Guarana.

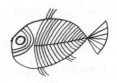

A year later he decided to institute a second test. There were eight subjects between the ages of 25 and 43. Before commencement of the study blood tests were taken to establish fibrinogen, cholesterol, HDL (high density lipoprotein) and sedimentation rate. The patients were all weighed and questioned as to their consumption of coffee on the day prior to the test beginning. All eight believed themselves to be in good health.

As in the previous experiment the dosage of Guarana was two capsules (500 mg each) of powdered Guarana. The first was taken on an empty stomach before breakfast and the second in the middle of the afternoon. The trial covered a three-month period and all the blood tests were repeated on the last day of the third month.

The fibrinogen level fell in five of the subjects by between 0.3 and 1.3 mmol/l; in the remaining three participants there was no increase or decrease in fibrinogen. The HDL measurement showed an increase ranging from 0.3 to 0.8 mmol/l in four of the volunteers, only one of whom also showed a drop in the fibrinogen level. One patient lost a total of 1.5 kg, another lost 3 kg and one gained 1 kg. The weight of the other five remained unchanged throughout the study. There was no change in their regular coffee consumption.

Six out of the eight reported an overall increase in their sense of energy, most specifically during the morning and the afternoon. Some of the participants had taken part in the previous trial and were positive that their overall feeling of increased energy was much more than when they took part in the short study.

Apart from the slightly looser stools reported by some of the participants in both studies, there were no observable side-effects or adverse reactions. This second test was not a double-blind study, its purpose being to establish any long-term effects of consuming a regular daily dose of Guarana.

Bo Netterstrom came to the conclusion that after this three-month trial to study the effects of taking Guarana over a longer period there was a fall in the fibrinogen levels in the blood. Furthermore there was a greater feeling of an energy boost than was experienced in the short study. This experiment does not 'prove' that Guarana reduces stress or generates energy. But most of the participants in both studies reported subjective feelings of more energy, and the findings of significant falls in fibrinogen levels – which are known to rise under situations of stress – go a long way to supporting the claims made for this plant by the rainforest Indians.

Guarana improves mood and performance

In an elegant little study, Reading Scientific Services Limited examined the effects of Guarana on both mood and performance in a group of subjects. They have been developing methods for assessing the effects of foods and food ingredients on human mood and performance, and now have a set of experimental tests which make it possible to assess and measure these effects and to compare the results of using different substances.

Their experimental format uses a series of computerised tasks which allow them to measure changes in both the speed and the accuracy with which subjects perform specific tasks. Before the programme the subject's base-line performance is identified. They then undertake the computerised tests, for which no previous computer skills are necessary.

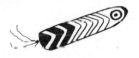

In this controlled study using Reading Scientific Services computerised tests, the comparative effects of Guarana and caffeine on both mood and performance on a group of volunteers were investigated. It was established that Guarana had strong and consistently positive effects on those taking part.

This experiment is of particular interest to me as there have been suggestions that the effects of Guarana are attributable to caffeine. Here we are able to see a clear demonstration that Guarana acts in a quite different way from caffeine and produces none of the undesirable side-effects of what is probably the world's most widely used stimulant drug.

Two levels of caffeine dosage were compared with the same dose of Guarana as before, and a control was established by using capsules of food-grade starch as a placebo. The subjects were given the high-dose caffeine, the low-dose caffeine, the Guarana or the placebo capsule on each of four test days. The participants were unaware of the contents of the capsules. The performance and mood of the

Figure 1: Effect of Guarana and caffeine on friendliness
Anatagonist/Friendly

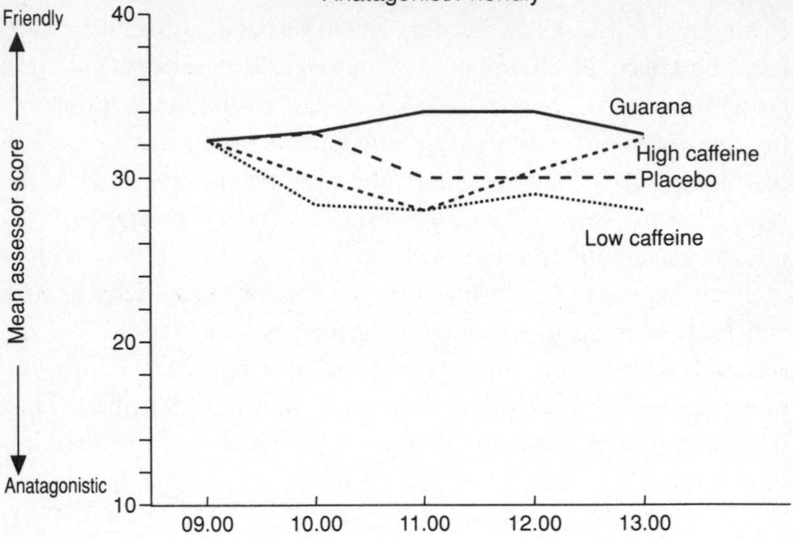

participants were measured over a four-hour period, following a base-line measurement before they were given the capsules. Each participant was given two capsules during the four-hour study period.

The effects of both caffeine and Guarana on the performance of a task designed to measure sustained attention were small; the doses of Guarana resulted in the fastest reaction times, but only by a small margin. In a test of hand–eye co-ordination a much greater divergence was shown between the four test capsules. Guarana improved the speed and to a lesser extent the accuracy. The high caffeine dose actually had an adverse effect in this test; in some instances participants on the high caffeine dose performed even less well than when taking the placebo.

Examination of the participants' mood revealed clear and consistent effects when assessing alertness, calmness and friendliness. The two charts show the effects of each of the capsules during a four-hour period averaged across the total number of participants. Figure 1 shows the mood of the participants on a scale varying from *drowsy* to *alert*. It is clearly shown that Guarana had extreme-

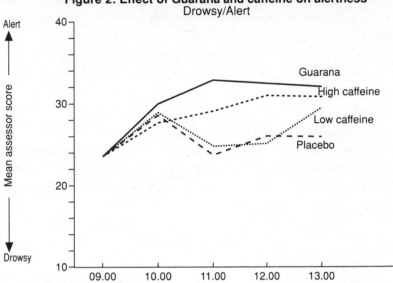

Figure 2: Effect of Guarana and caffeine on alertness
Drowsy/Alert

ly positive effects which were even greater than those achieved with the high dose of caffeine.

Figure 2 demonstrates the subjects' subjective and self-reported feelings of friendliness varying on the scale from *antagonistic* to *friendly*. Once again, you will see that there was a clear tendency for the participants to feel more friendly, sociable and outgoing when taking Guarana compared to when taking one of the other three capsules.

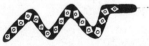

According to Reading Scientific Services, many of the differences between the substances are statistically significant, but they consider the importance of the results to lie in their consistency over a wide range of different measures. Their conclusion is that Guarana has a strong and consistent positive effect on reported mood and some positive effects on performance. Caffeine at a low dose had some positive effects, but at a high dose it had some negative effects on both mood and performance.

In my practice I regularly see patients who are caffeine abusers, even though most of them don't actually realise it. It is very disturbing to see people who have difficulty in sleeping and concentrating, who develop hand tremors, and who find themselves getting irritable, aggressive and sometimes even quite anti-social. They may already be drinking six or eight cups of coffee a day, and in an effort to overcome their difficulties increase it even more. They may be children or young teenagers whose parents wouldn't dream of giving them three cups of strong black coffee in the evening, but seem oblivious to the fact that they may be drinking vast amounts of cola drinks. Caffeine is present not only in coffee but also in cola drinks, chocolate and tea.

NEWSFLASH

From *Elle*, August 1990
In the Amazon Guarana and lambada are natural companions.
Both are fundamental sources of energy.DIS

There are many cases where by reducing the caffeine and by prescribing Guarana symptoms of agitation have disappeared in weeks.

Case history
Mr L.U., age 34, single, an economist

This man came to see me in the most appalling state. He was the institutional investment adviser for a huge banking organisation and the responsibilities of his job were beginning to overwhelm him. His main function was to advise managers of pension funds on the investment of their members' cash, work which he took extremely seriously as people's futures depended on his advice. In the wake of the Maxwell scandal and the alarmingly poor performance of some other pension funds, he had become riddled with anxiety. He feared that any mistakes which he might make would have devastating effects on the pensions of many thousands of ordinary hard-working people in years to come.

He had got into the habit of going to his office earlier and earlier each day and staying later every evening. Most of his weekends were spent scouring financial reports and using his computer to calculate long-term strategies. His sleep had become fitful and disturbed by bad dreams, he had lost a stone and a half in weight over the previous six months, and he looked terrible.

He had got himself locked into a self-fulfilling prophesy of doom and gloom, finding it increasingly more difficult to make decisions and losing all of his customary self-confidence and vitality. As a result of his appearance and the obvious changes in his demeanour clients who had always trusted him implicitly began to question his advice. This only served to magnify his feelings of insecurity.

By the time he got to me he was well down the slippery slope – his doctor had tried him on various sleeping pills, tranquillisers and anti-depressants, all of which, he claimed, turned him into a zombie. Just to keep himself going he was consuming vast amounts of coffee – up to twenty cups a day – and when things got really bad he was taking caffeine pills as well.

After several months at this level of caffeine consumption, it becomes extremely difficult to reduce the intake without suffering severe withdrawal effects. Violent headaches, tremors and deep depression are all likely side-effects. The effects on mood swings can also be quite alarming and even the normally amiable may turn aggressive.

With poor Mr L.U. we were faced with a complicated mix of problems: his own psychological fears, the established pattern of insomnia, a virtually constant state of depression, and the addiction to massive doses of caffeine and their resulting physical and behavioural side-effects. The first step was to begin a gradual reduction in his daily caffeine intake. He was advised to mix 25% of decaffeinated coffee with 75% normal coffee for the first two weeks. At the same time he was given a daily dose of 2 g of Guarana, one tablet of Genesis multi-vitamin and mineral preparation per day, and 250 IU of vitamin E daily.

This regime – combined with relaxation exercises, massage and aromatherapy – began the unwinding process. At the same time he was advised to improve his eating habits by eating a substantial breakfast of porridge or muesli, wholemeal toast, some protein in the form of an egg, some cheese or some fish, and a piece of fresh fruit. He was told he had to take an hour off in the middle of the day and get out of his office for a brisk twenty-minute walk and a sensible lunch. A good meal including plenty of vegetables and salads in the evening and at least three pints of water a day rounded off the dietary advice. After a fortnight the coffee mixture switched to 50:50 regular and decaffeinated, and by the fifth week the mixture was 75% decaffeinated to 25% regular.

By the end of two months the change was astounding. He gained three-quarters of a stone, he was getting five to six hours of sound sleep nightly, and the tremors and irritability had almost disappeared. By now he was drinking no more than half a dozen cups of the coffee mixture and substituting herbal teas for his other drinks. He was having regular sessions with a counsellor to resolve his fears regarding work and his self-confidence was growing daily. The regular 2 g of Guarana was a fixed item in his daily regime and the gentle, long-acting stimulus of this Brazilian herb carried him through his working days with none of the unwanted, unpleasant and damaging side-effects of vast amounts of caffeine.

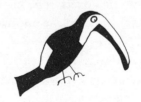

There is some confusion over the chemical nature of the compounds which seem to produce the stimulating effects of Guarana. The traditional theory is that the active ingredient is a tetramethyl xanthene rather than a trimethyl xanthene – caffeine. Both Henman in 1982 and Hildreth in 1989 maintained that guaranine is not identical to caffeine because it is a tetramethyl xanthene. It is also believed that the traditional Indian method of production by stone-grinding and sun-drying preserves the guaranine. It is claimed that guaranine is converted to caffeine during the highly commercial grinding and roasting processes employed by some industrial manufacturers.

A. R. Henman (1982), professor of ethnobotany at the University of Campinas (Unicamp), São Paulo, Brazil, also suggests that the slow release and long-term stimulating effects of Guarana occur as a result of other components of the seeds, specifically tannins and saponins. These slow down the rate at which guaranine dissolves in the digestive system and also the speed with which it is absorbed through the gut wall. Certainly my observations would confirm this. Patients given Guarana do not get the sudden rush of hyperactivity associated with caffeine, nor have I ever seen a patient with Guarana addiction. Addiction is common in heavy coffee drinkers. The trembling hands, poor sleep and irritability associated with caffeinism have never been seen by me – or to my knowledge reported in the literature – in relation to Guarana. This is of course my own simple observation and does not constitute a scientific double-blind study.

In 1993 P. J. Houghton of King's College, London, published a paper, together with Bempong and Steadman, in the *International Journal of Pharmacognosy*. In this paper the writers identified caffeine as the major xanthene present in Guarana through a series of experiments which failed to identify guaranine as a tetramethyl xanthene. According to their results, a standard dose of Guarana contains less than half the amount of caffeine than a cup of tea made with one teabag containing 2.5 g of leaf, and an even smaller percentage of the caffeine content of a cup of instant coffee made with 2.5 g of coffee powder. Even if one accepts that caffeine is present in Guarana, a dose would give you less than 20% of the amount of caffeine than an average cappuccino does.

In spite of their conviction that it is only the caffeine in Guarana that is effective, they conclude their paper by saying:

> The recommended doses of Guarana products do not
> contain as much caffeine as a cup of tea or instant coffee. If
> the stimulant effect observed is due to caffeine, it would
> therefore not be particularly noticeable except in the case of

individuals who were on a caffeine-free diet. Work is in progress on the nature of other constituents present in the seeds and their possible intrinsic stimulant activity or effect on caffeine release.

There have been other scientific evaluations attributing Guarana's effects to its caffeine content alone. These include a further study by Bempong and Houghton at King's College, London, which compared the rate of release of caffeine from capsules of Guarana with that from capsules containing an equivalent amount of caffeine. They studied the rate of absorption of caffeine through rat intestines and could demonstrate no difference in the release or uptake of caffeine from Guarana and preparations containing free caffeine.

No one would argue with the scientist who seeks to establish the precise way in which chemicals react with each other or with the human body; no one could argue with the researcher seeking after

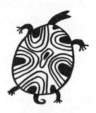

scientific truth; no one could argue with the pharmacologist or the physician determined to prove the safety of any preparation recommended for use as a medicament.

But I would argue with all of them when they try to apply the 'magic bullet' theory to the complex activities of plant medicines. There are countless illustrations of the way in which the natural combination of the chemical constituents of a plant is precisely the reason for its efficacy. It is equally true that when the supposed active principle is extracted from a complex natural structure, you can be left with a single chemical which is toxic although the original whole plant was both effective and safe. There is a naturally synergistic relationship between the components in many herbal extracts and it is this synergy which results in both the beneficial action and the lack of toxicity found when you consider Guarana.

We can glean a minute insight into the complexities of nature through the work of research scientists at the University of California, San Diego. Earlier in the book we have looked at the tragic fate of the Pacific yew, a tree previously believed to be useless, resulting in the eradication of 90% of examples of it from the American landscape. Now we know that this tree yields a substance which will treat advanced and otherwise non-responsive forms of cancer. There are no longer enough trees to supply the amount of this substance, taxol, that is needed. After years of work scientists are on the way to synthesising this substance, a task which they have described as massive. Two precursors of the taxane ring, which themselves both needed highly complex synthesis, produced only a 23% yield of taxane. Twenty-eight more steps were involved before the laboratory could produce taxol – something which nature does unaided.

Traditionally, plant medicines have depended on using an extract of the entire root, complete leaves, all of the fruits, seeds or nuts, the bark and sometimes the whole plant. The herbalist, the shaman, the medicine man and the village wise woman all work in this way. They never attempt to separate the different components of their extracts and I believe that it is a mistake to do so in today's scientific society. The commercial pressures to do so are enormous. There is no patent for whole plants – though the genetic engineers are trying to patent new varieties – so no pharmaceutical company can corner the market in a new plant medicine unless they isolate a specific constituent and patent the process, or play molecular roulette and produce a new substance.

The traditional explanation of the stimulating effects of Guarana is simple. The gently sun-dried and stone-ground seeds of Guarana contain a number of active substances, one of which is a caffeine-like chemical, tetramethyl xanthene. In industrial oven-roasting and crushing on hot steel rollers the tetramethyl xanthene is converted to trimethyl xanthene – caffeine. Theobromine and theophylline are also present, albeit in quite small amounts, but these have their own therapeutic values which will be discussed further on in this chapter. In Brazil this whole group of alkaloids is known as 'guaranine' and it is, I believe, the synergistic effects of this combination of chemicals that make Guarana such a valuable plant.

NEWSFLASH

From *The Sunday Times*, 12 April 1987

In the beginning there was ginseng. Then came royal jelly. Now the Brazilians have come up with Latin America's answer to executive stress, examination nerves and a lack-lustre love life.

It is Paullinia cupana, otherwise known as Brazilian Cocoa or Guarana Bread, the stone ground seeds of the berry found on the tropical climber Guarana plant.

The Indians, it is claimed, revere it as a potent aphrodisiac and energy booster. The Brazilians are so convinced of its power that they drink an estimated 2 million cups of Guarana tea a day.

Some of the scientific literature describes Guarana as the plant which provides the most caffeine of all, far more than the coffee bean, the cocoa bean or the tea leaf. While this may be true in terms of the percentage of caffeine – in that industrially prepared Guarana powder will yield between 3.5 and 4% by weight, which is about twice the yield of coffee and three times that of tea – this type of comparison is grossly misleading. The recommended daily dose of Guarana as a supplement or medicament is 1 g, but the amount of tea or coffee consumed in every cup is hugely more. If we compare the amount of caffeine in a 200 ml serving of various drinks with the amount in a daily dose of Guarana, we arrive at the following figures:

Coffee (brewed)	100–200 mg
Coffee (instant)	80–100 mg
Tea	70–100 mg
Cola drinks	55 mg
Guarana, daily dose	35 mg

Another consideration is the different way in which the constituents of tea and coffee dissolve. As both of these are water soluble they can be simply prepared by infusing with boiling water. The caffeine content is released into the water and starts to enter the bloodstream as soon as the tea or coffee is drunk. The resulting stimulation of the central nervous and circulatory system is virtually instantaneous.

Guarana behaves in an entirely different way. As the plant is a member of the *Sapindaceae* family – the soapwoods – all its tissues, but most especially the seeds, are rich in saponins, the natural oils and fats which abound in this family. Saponins are not water soluble and, consequently, traditionally prepared Guarana will not dissolve easily in boiling water or make a simple and quick infusion. The presence of these natural fats and oils interferes with the assimilation of the active components, resulting in a slower absorption rate and a much gentler, longer-lasting effect. Some reports describe the length of time for the absorption of all the xanthene from a 1 g dose of traditional Guarana as being up to six hours.

To sum up the caffeine argument, there is no doubt that there is caffeine in Guarana. There is also no doubt that clinical experience, a thousand years of use by the rainforest Indians and studies by western scientists dating back to the first written description in 1669 conclusively show that Guarana does not act in the same way as caffeine on the human body.

Whether or not the tetramethyl xanthene described by some early researchers exists, it is certain that the term 'guaranine' is suitable as an umbrella description of the whole group of chemicals which make Guarana such a fascinating plant to study and such a valuable plant to use therapeutically. It may be scientifically inaccurate, but it is clinically and practically of much more value than any other term. As we have already seen, it is a basic principle of herbal medicine that the effect of any single isolated component of a plant extract is not always the same as the effect of an extract from the whole plant. In fact this is seldom the case.

In various papers Henman has discussed the startling difference between the high caffeine content of Guarana and its mild long-lasting effects. He believes, in true herbalist's fashion, that there is a balance and counter-balance effect produced by the saponins in Guarana. Henman further states that:

> Little interest has been shown in examining the non-alkaloidal properties of Guarana which may well play an important part in the drug's pharmacology. It is probably both the nutritive value of these fatty compounds and the relative slowness which they afford to the absorption of the stimulant alkaloids, which together have given Guarana its reputation as a 'healthy' pick-me-up, and a sustaining food substitute during periods of voluntary or enforced fasting.

NEWSFLASH

From *Country Living*, November 1990

Renowned author and investigator of herbal medicines, Barbara Griggs writes:

Millions of Brazilians would be affronted by anyone doubting the powers of Guarana: to them it is an indispensable, all-purpose pick me up and general tonic. From the President downwards, everybody takes it.

Case history
Mrs S.G. – Guarana as a palliative during prolonged periods of restricted food intake

Mrs S.G. was 53 years old, grossly obese and suffering severe pain in her right hip. Examination and X-rays revealed advanced osteoarthritis in the hip joint and she was referred to an orthopaedic surgeon. Generally speaking, there is great reluctance to perform hip replacement surgery on patients as young as Mrs S.G., the early to mid-60s being the preferred age. In this case it was clear that she would soon be totally incapacitated, unable to care for her family or continue with her part-time employment. The surgeon said he was prepared to operate but not until she had lost five stones, reducing her weight from the current seventeen stone down to twelve.

She was desperate to have the operation and also desperate because she had struggled with her weight from her late teens. She had followed every diet, spent years going on and off to Weight-Watchers and had been prescribed every legal slimming pill. She had tried the slimming biscuits, the meal replacements, the diet meals, hypnosis, acupuncture and even group therapy – all to no avail. How was she going to lose the five stones needed to satisfy the surgeon?

The biggest problem she faced was severe exhaustion. As soon as her calorie intake was reduced she felt she just could not cope. Of course, the simple exertion of getting out of a chair and crossing the room was painful and required an enormous amount of energy in order to move her bulk. There was no question of trying crash diets or even 1,000-calorie-a-day diets, as she would never cope. On the other hand, it was essential to produce a rapid early weight loss in order to give her the encouragement she needed. We undertook a careful analysis of her diet and found that her perception of what she ate did not quite match up with the reality. She was consuming far too many calories from fats and sugars, and getting far too few calories from complex carbohydrates. Too much protein, not enough fibre, too many snacks and not enough fruit and vegetables were all compounded by an ever-increasing amount of time spent sitting as a result of the painful hip.

For two weeks Mrs S.G. was given 1 g of Guarana and a multi-vitamin and mineral pill each day. She started a programme of non-weight-bearing exercises which she could do lying on her bed or sitting in an armchair. Thanks to the support of her daughter, we managed to persuade her into the local swimming pool, where she joined an aquarobics class specifically designed for people with arthritis.

At the end of the two weeks she was already feeling slightly more energetic. Before even starting on the initial diet plan, she had lost four pounds. On Day 1 of the diet the dose of Guarana was doubled to 2 g and Mrs S.G. started on the regime which was to last for a month. The objective was to combine as much exercise as her physical condition allowed, a programme of healthy controlled eating at around 1,100 calories per day, a dose of Guarana to maintain energy levels and a vitamin pill to ensure sufficient nutrient intake. The estimated weight loss was a maximum of two to three pounds per week.

Here is the diet that Mrs S.G. followed for four weeks.

The Healthy Eating Plan

MONDAY

Breakfast:
Baked beans on toast with a grilled tomato; a cup of tea or coffee with semi-skimmed milk. Have either drink with breakfast every day.
Light meal:
A large portion of coleslaw made with red, white and green cabbage, carrots, sultanas, onion, apple, plain yoghurt, a little olive oil and a tablespoon of cider vinegar, with a small cup of cottage cheese and a piece of fresh fruit.
Main meal:
Chicken breast (skin removed) covered with a sliced courgette, thin strips of red pepper, a little garlic, the juice of a lemon, half a glass of dry white wine and quarter of a pint of vegetable stock (from a cube) cooked in a covered casserole for 30 minutes at 175°C/350°F/Gas

---

Mark 4, with carrots and parsnips mashed together. A baked apple (cooked in the oven at the same time). Remove the core, cut off the bottom quarter, put the rest back in the centre and fill with 1 oz ground almonds mixed with orange juice, sprinkled with a little cinnamon and nutmeg.

TUESDAY

Breakfast:
Porridge made with half-water, half-skimmed milk, a slice of wholemeal toast with a little butter and honey.

Light meal:
A large bowl of vegetable, bean and barley soup – for 6 large portions use 1 oz pot barley, 1½ pints water, 4 sliced carrots, 1 chopped turnip, 2 sliced leeks, 2 sticks celery, 1 chopped onion, 1 dsp tomato purée, black pepper; bring them to the boil and simmer for 45 minutes. Add a can of kidney, butter, haricot or any other sort of beans, cook for another 5 minutes. Serve with a green salad with oil and vinegar dressing.

Main meal:
Any grilled fish with a green vegetable followed by some soft cheese with a large stick of crunchy celery.

WEDNESDAY

Breakfast:
Half a grapefruit, 2 poached eggs, 2 grilled tomatoes.

Light meal:
2 or 3 large flat mushrooms or a good handful of button mushrooms fried in a little butter very gently in a covered pan for about 15 minutes on wholemeal toast with a salad.

Main meal:
Grilled lamb chops with most of the fat removed, peas and carrots; a portion of dried fruits soaked and served with low fat natural yoghurt mixed with a pinch of cinnamon, grated lemon rind and a teaspoon of honey.

THURSDAY

Breakfast:
A mixture of an orange, an apple and a pear sliced into a bowl with a carton of natural yoghurt and a teaspoonful of honey.

Light meal:
A sandwich of wholemeal bread without butter, a mashed banana, a couple of chopped-up dates, a squeeze of lemon juice and a sprinkle of any chopped nuts. A fresh pear and a few grapes.

Main meal:
Chicken cooked any way you like except fried, with at least two different vegetables. Chopped ready-to-eat Californian prunes and apricots soaked in the juice of a lemon, an orange, a tablespoon of brandy, half a teaspoon of sugar.

FRIDAY

Breakfast:
2 boiled eggs, 2 slices of wholemeal toast spread very thinly with butter.

Light meal:
A bowl of bean and barley soup (left over from Tuesday) with a wholemeal roll.

Main meal:
Put a fillet of hake or cod on a finely chopped onion, tomato and garlic mixture and then on a large piece of cooking foil, sprinkle more of the mixture on top of the fish, season with pepper and a little olive oil. Wrap the foil into a parcel, bake at 200°C/400°F/Gas Mark 6 for 20 minutes. Serve with a salad of watercress, orange segments and chicory. A piece of soft cheese (Brie, Camembert etc.) and a bunch of grapes.

SATURDAY

Breakfast:
As much fresh fruit as you like.

Light meal:
Italian toast — bruschetta. Toast a thick slice of coarse wholemeal bread until lightly brown on both sides. Rub one side with a cut clove of garlic, dribble on a little olive oil and pile with thin slices of fresh tomato — a wonderful snack for any time of the day or night.

Main meal:
Chicken, beef or lamb casserole — remove skin and fat, cut into cubes, seal for a few seconds in hot oil, remove the meat with a slotted spoon, add onion, garlic and celery; continue cooking until soft but not brown, add vegetable stock (from cube) with diced parsnip, carrot, swede, leek, turnip, potato; return meat to the mixture, cover tightly and cook at 180°C/350°F/Gas Mark 4 for 1–1½ hours till meat is tender. 2 tangerines in segments with a small carton of fromage frais and a teaspoon of honey.

SUNDAY

Breakfast:
2 slices of wholemeal toast with a little butter and honey. A glass of fresh orange juice.

Light meal:
Green pasta and tuna fish. While the pasta is cooking put 4 coarsely chopped spring onions including the green tops into a frying pan with a little oil. When they're soft add a small can of drained tuna and stir until warm but not cooked. Drain the pasta, return to the saucepan, mix in the tuna and spring onions and serve. A piece of fresh fruit.

Main meal:
Stir-fry lamb. Remove all fat from the meat and cut into thin strips. Put in a shallow dish with 1 tablespoon olive oil, 2 teaspoons soya sauce, 1 tablespoon dry sherry; leave to marinate for 30 minutes. Then in a wok or thick-bottomed frying pan heat some olive oil, add the lamb and some of the marinade, stirring vigorously for 3 minutes. Add a small leek thinly sliced lengthways, stir for another 2 minutes, then add a chopped spring onion, a chopped clove of garlic and a little freshly grated ginger and cook for another 3 minutes. Serve with a tomato and onion salad. Half a small melon.

Mrs S.G. was told to drink at least three pints of fluid each day – water, diluted unsweetened fruit juices and some tea and coffee. She was allowed one glass of wine or half a pint of beer or one pub measure of spirits each day as well.

This seven days of delicious healthy eating was designed to be enjoyed. It is not a slimming diet but an eating plan to help bring about long-term changes in eating patterns and to encourage gradual weight loss rather than dramatic results.

At the end of the first week she had lost two-and-a-half pounds, but in the second week her weight remained static. During Week 3 she was delighted as she had shed just under seven pounds, and another four pounds came off in Week 4 – almost a stone in just one month. After this initial period she was allowed to be a little more flexible in her eating, but was still weighed at the end of each week. For the first time in her life Mrs S.G. was able to control her food intake, reduce her overall calorie consumption and do without the endless nibbles which had contributed to her obesity. Thanks to the Guarana there was no fatigue and as the weight reduced she developed a much greater sense of her own worth and an enhanced feeling of well-being.

Just carrying less weight about was a major factor in her fatigue reduction and also enabled her to be gradually more active as the decrease in weight loading on her damaged hip produced a noticeable reduction in her pain and immobility. She reached her target weight of twelve stone by the end of the fourth month and proudly presented herself to the surgeon. He was so delighted that he put her on the 'urgent' list and within five weeks she had her operation. Two years later she was a fit and active woman, still enjoying her new-found way of eating, maintaining her weight at around twelve stone and still to be found in the local swimming pool at least three times a week.

NEWSFLASH

From *The Guardian*, Friday 12 June 1992
Earth Summit
Bleary eyed delegates who have been working on the final texts through the night are often to be found asleep during press conferences. Tranquillisers and vitamin pills have run out at the Rio Centre pharmacy. Some delegates are said to be relying on Guarana, an Amazon stimulant.

In April 1980 Professor A. R. Henman, one of the world's greatest authorities on native medicinal plants and their cultivation, presented a paper to the Annual General Meeting of the Economic and Medicinal Plants Research Association held at Downing College, Cambridge. This paper was subsequently updated and published by Henman in the *Journal of Ethnopharmacology*, 6 (1982). The paper is an eloquent plea for the proper cultivation and use of Guarana, a plant in which Henman sees one possible source of salvation for many of the problems that beset the Amazon rainforest.

Henman is deeply concerned that the main use of Guarana in recent decades has been as a flavouring agent and a source of caffeine for the soft drinks industry. He maintains that there are not only commercial but also serious medical reasons for encouraging and investigating the traditional methods of production and the reasons for using the seeds of the Guarana. Not only does the traditional preparation provide the stimulating effects described above, but it also has prophylactic properties and there is a possibility that it will prove its worth in the treatment of a number of specific health problems.

Henman points out that the very earliest accounts of this medicine show how highly it was regarded by the early settlers as well as by the indigenous Indians of the Amazon basin. Fasting was an important religious practice in many of the tribes, especially during pregnancy or after bereavement. Apparently during these magical periods the Indians' food consumption was restricted to manioc flour and flying ants. However, they were allowed to consume unlimited amounts of Guarana, which certainly helped them through long periods of very restricted eating.

From the very first writings about Guarana, in which the Jesuit missionary Bettendorf described in 1669 how the Indians drank Guarana tea as a part of their daily ritual, he noted their belief in its value as a treatment for headaches, fevers and cramps as well as for its diuretic effect. By the mid-1700s its use was widespread amongst the local European population. From the bishop down, the settlers found it was the best of all treatments for the recurrent diarrhoea from which they suffered and was also a wonderful aid to coping with the very high humidity and temperature in the tropical rainforest.

In 1826 the botanist von Martius sent samples of Guarana to his brother, who was the first to isolate the crystalline substance which he named 'guaranine'. Unusually large amounts of theobromine and theophylline were also found, together with around 6% of tannin. One exciting area highlighted by Henman is that of Guarana as a substitute for coffee and tea – especially for people suffering from heart and circulatory disease, for whom large intakes of caffeine are generally contra-indicated. In this paper he was particularly concerned about the lack of interest in the non-alkaloid properties of Guarana, especially the saponins. He cites work by the nineteenth-century German chemist Peckholt, who isolated a specific saponin called timbonine which has a similar chemical structure to the timbo fish poisons widely used by the Amazon Indians. Henman states in this paper:

> This would seem to be a grave oversight, particularly in the
> light of recent research into the therapeutic properties of

ginseng and other Old World stimulants which have demonstrated clearly that the pharmacological activity of such plants is due mainly to their saponin contents.

In August 1989 a fascinating patent application was submitted to the US Patent Office. The patent applied for was for a method of preparing a Guarana seed extract capable of inhibiting platelet aggregation in mammalian blood. Why was this so fascinating? Because in simple terms the inventor had found a way of using Guarana to prevent the formation of blood clots and to help in the breakdown of clots which have already formed. The rainforest Indians' claims that Guarana could 'thin the blood' were obviously more than just old wives' tales.

According to the patent application:

Blood platelets are small cells present in large numbers in mammalian blood and are vital in arresting bleeding by aggregating to form a platelet plug. When bleeding does not occur, internal injury to a blood vessel wall may cause formation of a platelet plug which is called a thrombus. Thrombus formation may block the flow of blood to an organ and cause infarction, a condition termed thrombosis. Thrombosis is considered to be a contributive cause to strokes, pulmonary embolisms, and myocardial infarctions. It is thus believed that ability to inhibit platelet aggregation and to deaggregate platelet aggregates would be of great benefit in reducing the adverse effects of thrombotic episodes.

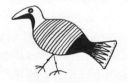

The principal object of the extraction process is to provide a composition which has no apparent undesirable side-effects, and has the ability to prevent blood clots from forming and to break down clots which may have already formed.

The inventor applying for this patent was Professor Ravi Subbiah. Together with his colleagues Bhadra and Agarwal at the Department of Internal Medicine, University of Cincinnati Medical Center, Cincinnati, Ohio, he published the final report on their studies on the anti-platelet aggregatory factors in the Brazilian herb Guarana (*Paullinia cupana*) on 1 July 1992. Subbiah and his team were intrigued by native claims that Guarana had some thinning effects on blood. In previous studies which Subbiah published in 1983 and in his patent application in 1989, he had demonstrated that the traditionally produced extracts of Guarana seeds did in fact reduce the speed with which blood platelets clumped together in the test tube as well as in the living body. What really excited the researchers was the way in which Guarana could deaggregate or unscramble already clotted platelets. This property was unlike any other platelet-active drugs, which only prevented these cells from clotting together and were of little use where clotting had already taken place.

In the 1992 study, blood was taken from human volunteers or from the blood bank and subjected to a range of tests designed to investigate the anti-clotting activity of Guarana on normal blood and on samples which had been treated with standardised clotting agents. Even when the methyl xanthines were removed from the Guarana extract, the resulting product remained as effective as the original in terms of its anti-platelet aggregatory properties.

Further confirmation of this dramatic benefit from Guarana was provided in a paper published in the *Brazilian Journal of Medical Biological Research*. S. P. Bydlowski – previously assistant to Professor Subbiah in Cincinnati, where the original research was done – together with colleagues D'amico and Chamone, reported on their continuing research into the anti-clotting mechanism of Guarana at the Faculty of Medicine of the University of São Paulo in Brazil. Having established that Guarana extract has a specific anti-clotting action on blood platelets, they attempted to identify the active compound in Guarana that was so powerfully active.

They separated the crude extract to remove the xanthenes and nicotinic acid which might have been responsible for the anti-

clotting action. While the xanthenes appear to be partially responsible for this beneficial effect, they found strong evidence for the
presence of other constituents which were part of the original
complete extract of Guarana and also had powerful anti-clotting
properties. Once again we see a convincing argument for the traditional herbalist's view that the value of the whole plant is always
greater than the sum of its individual constituents.

Even simple anti-clotting drugs like aspirin have side-effects and
are not tolerated by all patients. Asthmatics in particular may have
difficulties with aspirin and it is common for this drug to cause
digestive upsets, stomach ulcers and intestinal bleeding. Those in
need of anti-coagulant therapy are frequently required to be on
anti-clotting medication for long periods of time, which increases
the risk of side-effects. These studies, carried out with samples of
Guarana powder supplied by Rio Trading of Brighton, England,
open up an exciting new therapeutic avenue.

So far there is no evidence of adverse side-effects – the plant has
been in regular use by millions of people for thousands of years –
or of unwanted interactions with other medicines. Obviously until
further research is done patients in life-threatening situations will
still need to be prescribed the more powerful pharmaceutical drugs.
In these cases the risks of the drugs are far outweighed by the benefits. But there is no doubt in my mind that a regular daily dose of
Guarana should be a routine preventative step.

It is really important to get an idea of the huge impact which this
research could have worldwide. In 1991 at the American College of
Cardiology meeting, the preliminary results of a study with staggering implications were announced for the first time. This
research took the form of the largest meta-analysis (a study of all
the previous studies) ever undertaken. The results showed that a

modest dose of aspirin taken every day produced a 25% reduction in heart attacks, strokes and death in patients already suffering from some form of heart and circulatory illness.

In real terms that means the possible prevention of seven thousand premature deaths each year just in the UK and a hundred thousand worldwide.

Until then it was thought that this type of anti-platelet treatment was only of value in very specific groups of patients, such as those who had already sustained a stroke or heart attack. But the ground-breaking new work broadened the value of this therapy to include definite reductions in fatal heart attacks and strokes, equal benefits for women and for men, benefits for a much wider range of high-risk patients, and benefits in all high-risk patients no matter what their age or sex – even those suffering from diabetes or high blood-pressure.

Aspirin is cheap and easily available but all the evidence to date shows that Guarana may be just as effective and may lack the side-effects of aspirin.

There are many people at slight risk, those with just above normal blood-pressure, with slightly raised cholesterol levels, or with a close family history of blood-clotting disorders or heart disease. For all of these Guarana is a must. Even for the fittest amongst us, prevention is better than cure.

The natural buzz of Brazil – is it all in the mind?

We have already seen how Guarana improves psychological performance, but now we hear that young people have taken Guarana to their hearts. This is especially true amongst the frequenters of the discos, dance clubs and raves in England and America. In London, Leeds and Liverpool; in New York, New Orleans and Nashville; these energetic enthusiasts are turning away from booze and getting their kicks and the energy to dance away the night from Guarana. As the market for this rainforest remedy expands so we are seeing the arrival of the Guarana-flavoured Brazilian-type fizzy drinks as an alternative to the ubiquitous Coke, vials of concentrated liquid extract – a potent jungle juice if ever there was one – and capsules made from traditionally prepared Guarana seed. In fact now you can even get your buzz from Guarana chewing gum. But is it all in the mind?

Not according to Yoshinori Sato, head of the Japanese Central Research Laboratory, and his colleagues Masatoshi Terazawa, Joki Kinuma and Shichigoro Tezuka, who conducted the most fascinating series of studies on the drowsiness-prevention powers of chewing gum containing an extract of Guarana. No, you are not reading this on April Fools' Day – or even if you are, this is not a joke – the subject may seem flippant but the results have far-reaching consequences of considerable value.

These Japanese gentlemen have suggested that as society gets more complex the public is demanding more individual and diversified products; products which could not grow, thrive or survive simply by using conventional new product development techniques. The demands of today's society are more sophisticated and people no longer accept the same old goods in a package that says 'new' or 'improved'. One of the problems which they have addressed is that of drowsiness. They suggest that more and more people in our complex society struggle against this difficulty in order to achieve high levels of socioeconomic success and job satisfaction, and to maintain concentration at high levels over long hours.

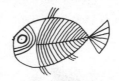

They single out for particular attention people driving long distances; shift workers who spend many hours monitoring sophisticated plant in the nuclear, chemical and energy-producing industries; those in the fire, hospital and police services; and do not forget students burning the midnight oil while preparing for examinations and falling asleep during the next day's lectures. In many of these situations not only are the individuals themselves at risk, but the effects on the public at large could be catastrophic if any of them nod of at the wrong moment. As they were already involved in the chewing gum industry, the Japanese team decided to combine their expertise with the tribal knowledge of the rainforest Indians, who have continuously credited Guarana with being a powerful and long-lasting stimulant.

What is drowsiness?

Drowsiness or fatigue is the state of mind and body that normally occurs before sleep. It causes gradual deterioration of performance as time passes. In this state you slow down, make silly mistakes and feel increasingly tired. At the extremes of drowsiness, when you are fighting to keep your eyes open and your brain functioning, there will be disruption of your powers of reasoning, deduction and judgement and it is highly likely that you will experience abnormal perception, such as hallucinations. Everyone knows that the most frequent cause of drowsiness and fatigue is lack of sleep. It is easy to show with simple experiments that one night of missed sleep or a couple of consecutive nights with only four or five hours will result in a measurable reduction in the ability to perform simple tasks. There is no doubt that some people are able to function at their peak even though they are deprived of the amount of normal sleep that most of us mere mortals would consider essential. There is a long history of short sleepers being the great doers of this world – Churchill, Napoleon, Ghengis Khan, Alexander the Great and even Lady Thatcher are examples.

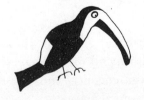

There are others whose very high level of motivation, be it geared to the performance of their duty or their sense of survival, enables them to function much better than is average on small amounts of sleep. Even the soldier in battle, the intrepid explorer in the most dangerous of situations and the doctor on duty for excessive hours in a major casualty department will not function at their best after a night of missed sleep, though they themselves may not always be aware of their shortcomings.

How Guarana fights fatigue at the wheel

As Sato and his colleagues had already looked at the links between drowsiness, driving and chewing gum, they decided to put Guarana to the test in the same way. As fatigue creeps up, performance begins to slow down and loss of concentration, forgetfulness and minor errors creep in to the behaviour pattern. Nearly always the individual is not in the slightest aware of what is happening. This does not matter much at home or in the office, but when the sufferer is transposed to the driving seat of a packed rush-hour bus, an express train, a 45-ton lorry or a car speeding down the motorway, then there is an accident waiting to happen.

A wide-awake and fully alert driver instantly absorbs, analyses and reacts to a variety of information: the speed of the car, road conditions, the distance from other vehicles, the child playing on the pavement, the school bus pulling in to the kerb, visibility and the performance of the vehicle being driven. The driver is then able to co-ordinate his or her responses in exactly the right sequence, mentally calculating braking distances and clearance tolerance, and predicting the behaviour of other road users. The drowsy driver will rivet his or her attention on one factor, which may be holding position between the white lines in the middle lane of the motorway, and exclude from his or her thought processes all consideration of other road hazards. The drowsy driver may complete whole sections of a journey without remembering the route that has been followed.

The drowsy driver is also much more likely to experience distortions of perception; trees appear to walk across the road, a pool of moonlight becomes a flood, a hundred yards look like twenty and twenty yards may appear to be a hundred. Many accidents occur when the drowsy driver takes avoiding action and swerves to miss a non-existent obstruction in the road. In the worst situation the driver finally falls asleep at the wheel and disaster follows.

All kinds of mechanical devices have been tried to alert drivers to this danger. Examples are buzzers or vibrating mechanisms which are triggered by the head nodding; advice to open the windows, take a break and walk around; encouragement to take a break and sleep, or to drink lots of black coffee; and even playing very loud music. The truth is that the drowsy driver is a dangerous driver and should not be on the road.

The Japanese researchers had already studied the arousal effect of chewing. In collaboration with the Japanese Transport Medicine Foundation they were able to determine how much the brain stem, and through it the cerebral cortex, could be stimulated by measuring brainwaves and the frequency of blinking in car drivers. What they investigated were the mechanical and psychological benefits of chewing and the effect of adding strong flavours to the chewing gum. Their initial studies produced some fascinating observations.

1. There is a significant relationship between the mechanical act of chewing and the prevention of drowsiness.
2. When they compared the effects of chewing gum, sweets and toffee they found that gum was much more effective than the others.
3. They found a positive psychological effect as the drivers had high expectations of the stimulating benefits that chewing gum would have in preventing drowsiness.
4. The stimulation of brainwaves was greatest when the drivers were given chewing gum with a strong mint flavour.
5. Measurements of the electrical reactions in the skin showed the greatest mental stimulation when chewing mint gum.

There is a fundamental difference between eating a piece of chocolate, a sweet or a toffee, and chewing gum. Ordinary confectionary is soon chewed and swallowed and, whilst this may produce a temporary rise in blood-sugar levels, it does not provide the continuing mechanical stimulation to the brain stem that is observed as a result of repeated chewing. The next step was to establish whether adding the known anti-fatigue benefits of Guarana to the chewing gum would enhance its effectiveness by providing a chemical as well as a mechanical stimulus.

Once again our researchers worked together with the Transport Medicine Research Foundation, using a selection of substances to compare the relative physiological effects on brainwaves, heart rate, breathing rate and eye flicks and the psychological effects on attentiveness. A placebo chewing gum, unflavoured and without Guarana, was tested against a mint-flavoured Guarana gum, a coffee-flavoured Guarana gum and three commercially available preparations marketed for the prevention of drowsiness. Preparation A was a tablet containing caffeine as its main ingredient. Preparation B was a mint sweet containing menthol, and preparation C was a different brand of mint sweet.

The placebo gum, used as the control, produced a mild stimulating effect through the mechanical stimulus of chewing but it was noticeably less effective than either of the Guarana gums. The mint candy B produced considerable arousal effects initially, but these receded rapidly once the sweet had been eaten. Product C was similar to B, but the effect was slightly longer lasting. The mint-flavoured Guarana gum produced immediate stimulation, first through the chewing action and secondly as a result of the strong mint flavour. The initial stimulus continued for around thirty-five to forty minutes, after which the effect began to fall off, at which time the pharmacological stimulus from the Guarana extract came into play.

The combination of chewing, mint flavour and Guarana produced a state of heightened awareness and diminished drowsiness dramatically above the initial resting state and this beneficial phase was maintained for over sixty minutes. The arousal curve lasted just over seventy minutes after the initial chewing of the mint Guarana gum before returning to the starting level. The coffee-flavoured

Guarana gum produced a similar result but the overall level of stimulus, though still significantly better than the placebo gum, was slightly less than that of the mint gum.

Sato and his colleagues concluded that the mint-flavoured Guarana gum combines three different functions which are of great value in combating drowsiness. Initially there is the mechanical stimulus of chewing accompanied by the rapid action of the mint flavour as a brain arouser, and this is followed by the slower-acting but much longer-lasting effect of the Guarana extract.

Recent evidence has shown that chewing gum after meals is a powerful protection against dental decay. If you chew Guarana gum you not only protect your teeth. If you are driving, especially at night, you could be protecting your life, your passengers' lives and those of innocent bystanders.

Migraine and tension headaches

One of the most frequently reported benefits of Guarana is its value in the relief of migraine and tension headaches. Guarana is described by herbalists as being both an 'adaptogen' and a 'nervine'. These are terms not likely to be familiar to your corner pharmacist. The term 'adaptogen' is quite new in the European herbal field, though it is one of the cornerstones of the holistic approach of Chinese and other eastern schools of healing. The adaptogen has the ability to improve the way in which the body adapts to changes in its own homeostasis – that is, the internal balance which keeps the body's machinery working in harmony.

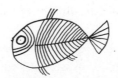

By functioning in this way Guarana is able to fend off the total collapse which looms as the result of excessive stresses, poor lifestyle, lack of sleep and the variety of emotional traumas which we accept as the norm in our frenetic twentieth-century-style of day-to-day living. Research points to the adaptogen raising the base-line level of the body's natural immune defence mechanism, possibly by stimulating the adrenal glands, and so protecting the individual from the secondary damage caused by stress.

The nervine is described as having a universally beneficial effect on the body's nervous system. It may seem a bit far fetched to suggest that any plant could have such a wide reaching and important effect on any of the body's systems, but it is a fact that many plants have precisely this ability, as sedatives, tonics or stimulants to the nervous system.

The combined adaptogen and nervine effects of Guarana explain many of its successful uses, but none so clearly as its value as a remedy for migraines and tension headaches. Both the American and the British *Pharmacopoeia* used to list this as the prime medical use of the Brazilian plant. Although there may be many different triggers for an attack of migraine – hormone changes, adverse food reactions, light, noise, heat, fatigue, low blood sugar, hunger, thirst, or even alcohol – underlying them all is a nervous reaction which allows these multiple factors to cause an attack of migraine.

The same is true of tension headaches, which may kick off with bad posture at work, tension when driving, fatigue, the wrong type of bed or pillow, occupational stresses linked to repetitive movements or poor working positions, or badly designed seats whether at work, home or in the car. Add to these physical and mechanical tensions the additional problems of anxiety, rush and stress and the headache becomes virtually inevitable.

The answer is often Guarana.

Case history
Miss C.B., age 22, trainee manager in a foodstore group

This charming and delightful young woman is poised on the threshold of a managerial career in the food retailing industry. She left university with an excellent 2.1 degree. She had suffered the occasional migraine – usually associated with her periods – while she was a student, but within three months they had increased to the point of almost wrecking her life. She was getting two or three attacks every week, some of them lasting a full twenty-four hours and leaving her like a wrung-out dishcloth the following day. Her employers were very understanding and did not put extra pressures on her because of her problem, but she became more and more stressed. She was extremely ambitious and a conscientious perfectionist and missing time from work and letting her colleagues and the bosses down was a major source of anxiety to her.

Her social life had ground to a complete standstill. She refused all invitations. Never knowing when the migraine would strike, she hated the thought of cancelling arrangements and inconveniencing her friends. By the time I saw this poor young woman she had tried all the orthodox drugs, none of which had proved particularly successful. She'd been seen by neurologists, she'd been put on the Pill, and at the suggestion of a friend of the family she had consulted a so-called allergy specialist, who used a pendulum to diagnose that she was allergic to almost everything. She then followed such a rigid exclusion diet that she became extremely thin, very anaemic and seriously deficient in many of the essential vitamins and minerals. Needless to say, as she got weaker and more worried the migraines became worse and more frequent.

The first thing we did was to sit down and talk at length about her eating pattern. She was given a sensible eating plan of high-quality and nutrient-dense foods – excluding the most likely migraine triggers: cheese, chocolate, oranges, alcohol and coffee. She was instructed to eat some food every two hours to maintain her blood-sugar level on an even keel, and to drink four pints of water every day to keep her kidneys working at their peak level. She was given high-dose vitamin and mineral supplements to restore her nutritional status to normal in as short as possible a time. Massage, osteopathic treatment, acupuncture and relaxation exercises were all included in her regime. In addition to all this, she was started immediately on 1 g of Guarana every morning, and ½ g at lunch-time. A further ½ g was to be taken with two large glasses of cold water at the first sign of a migraine developing.

Within two weeks the nervine and adaptogen properties of Guarana started to do their work. In conjunction with all the other treatments the Guarana had set her off on the road to recovery. By the second month she was getting a mild attack of migraine on the day before her period was due – still bad enough for her to have to stay at home. After four months these were reduced to mild headaches which did not prevent her from enjoying work or social activities. By the end of a year she was virtually headache-free, had not missed a day of work in six months, was looking wonderful and taking care of her own health. Of course, she was still taking two capsules of Guarana every morning.

With this form of complex holistic approach to health problems, it is not always possible to know exactly which bit of which therapy might be doing the most good. I can only say that the delightful Miss C.B. is one of many patients who have responded better to their migraine treatment since I began using Guarana as part of an overall scheme.

It never ceases to amaze me that some drugs and some surgical procedures acquire instant recognition from the medical profession – the editor of the *British Medical Journal* recently told me that little in the publication is the truth; read this week's issue in twenty years' time and very little of today's perceived wisdom will still be current. It will be shown later that it was at best ineffective, and at worst seriously harmful to patients. The other side of the coin is the vast treasure trove of useful knowledge locked away in dusty old tomes, in research institutes, and in university archives. I cannot resist giving you the following example:

> Guarana – Medical Properties and Uses. The effects of
> Guarana upon the system are chiefly those of its alkaloid,
> although it contains enough tannin to have an appreciable
> influence. It is habitually employed by the Indians, either
> mixed with articles of diet, as with cassava or chocolate, or
> in the form of a drink, prepared by scraping it, and suspend-
> ing the powder in sweetened water, precisely as other

nations use teas, coffees, etc. It is also considered by the Indians useful in the prevention and cure of bowel complaints. Doctor Gavrelle, who was at one time physician to Dom Pedro, in Brazil, and there became acquainted with the virtues of this medicine, called the attention of the profession to it some years since in France. He had found it advantageous in the diarrhoea, sick headache, and as a tonic. It has since been employed in various affections, but is now chiefly used in migraine, administered when the attack is developing. It may be given in powder, in the quantity of one or two drachms [3.9 to 7.8 g], or the fluid extract may be substituted. (From *The Dispensatory of the United States of America*, 17th Edition, Philadelphia, 1894)

The Guarana Project

I have already mentioned the dedicated and pioneering efforts of Denise and Graeme Lewis, Ben Nash and their company, Rio Trading. As a result of their investigations and, I believe, much more as a result of their total dedication to improving the lot of the rainforest dwellers and all mankind, they have now launched an exciting new initiative.

An outcome of their existing research programme and the encouraging developments which are already growing out of it, is that they have formed a separate company, Rio Pharmaceuticals Limited, to take over the existing work and to look for new scientific initiatives in the rainforest. This enterprise will be headed by scientific director David Williams, a scientist with thirty-five years' experience in the pharmaceutical field. He will be leading the Guarana Project, among others.

Graeme Lewis told me that Rio Pharmaceuticals intend to identify further projects to follow the Guarana research programme, and that they plan to develop a range of plant-based medicines which will lead the way into the next century. He said:

> It is well known that the medicinal potential of Amazon plants is vast and we are determined to be in the forefront of research. But Rio's commitment to the peoples and cultures of the Amazon Basin will ensure that proper returns are made to those who carry the herbal and medical knowledge, and whose way of life in the rainforest must be preserved.

8 Lapacho, Pfaffia, Catuaba and Stevia

'If I am right, vegetable soup offers more promise in reducing mortality from cancer than do present medicines.'

James Duke, ethnobotanist,
US Department of Agriculture

There are many thousands of plants growing in the lushness of the Brazilian rainforest, some of which we already know to have powerful medicinal activity. Some of these are already available as commercial products and are, I am sure, just the tip of the iceberg. On-going research will certainly produce the information that will lead us to even greater discoveries of nature's bounty. There are plants which may hold the key to the treatment of HIV and the prevention of AIDS, plants which will certainly play a major role in the treatment of cancers, plants which are natural anti-inflammatories and will benefit those with joint disease and skin conditions, and plants which will yield natural hormone-like substances for the treatment of glandular disorders.

Here we look at just a few of the gifts from the rainforest that we already have knowledge of.

Lapacho

Otherwise known as Pau d'Arco, Ipe Roxo or Taheebo, this native medicine is made from the inner bark of a large rainforest tree, the

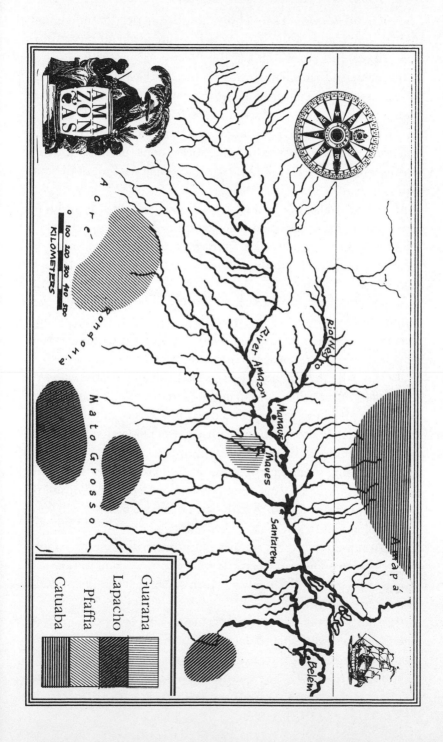

Tabebuia avellenedae. Throughout South America the inhabitants use the inner layer of the bark, which is shredded and made into a form of tea. It is taken to boost the effectiveness of the body's own immune-defence mechanisms. The Indians have used this traditional remedy for centuries as the treatment for asthma, diabetes, bronchitis, infections and even some forms of cancer. Although much of the evidence is anecdotal and there has to date been little scientific research, that which has been done promises exciting results which yet again reinforce the traditional wisdom of the rain-forest Indians.

The Argentinian botanist Dr Meyer spent the last years of his life trying to persuade the scientific establishment that Lapacho was a plant of great potential value. Sadly, he died a frustrated man.

As far back as 1882 one of the constituents was isolated by Paterno and identified as lapachol, an anti-microbial and anti-tumour chemical. Dr Paul Lee, writing in the magazine *Total Health* in December 1991, states that Lapacho has effects on both cancer and candida infections. What is more, it is useful as a remedy for colds, flu, fevers, infections and even lupus.

Research by the Japanese doctors Ikekawa and Yoshikawa at the National Cancer Centre in Japan, has demonstrated an anti-cancer substance present in the Lapacho tree which has what they describe as 'potent' anti-cancer action against leukaemia and some specific malignant tumours such as stomach cancer. One piece of research with surprising results, carried out at the University of São Paulo, came about in the process of extracting pure lapachol. During the experiment it was found that the crude extract had a much more powerful antibiotic effect than the purified end product, leading to the assumption that there are other anti-bacterial substances in this amazing plant. The crude extracts were effective against a very wide range of bacterial and fungal organisms including *Candida albicans* – the cause of thrush.

In another series of experiments at the University of São Paulo, the researchers were able to demonstrate that Lapacho has extremely low toxicity, but at the same time possesses valuable anti-inflammatory properties. These experiments were extended to a group of patients suffering from a variety of different cancers. Here the results showed low toxicity and definite anti-tumour activity in liver, breast and prostate cancers. Lapacho also appeared to reduce

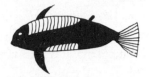

the pain level in most of the patients studied.

At the Department of Biological Chemistry at Harvard Medical School, Boothman and Pardee conducted another fascinating study published in the *Proceedings of the National Academy of Science, USA, July 1989*. Their work involved creating cancerous changes in cell cultures using radiation in the form of X-rays. What they were able to demonstrate was that treating the cells with β-lapachone after they had been irradiated produced an eight-fold reduction in the number of damaged cells. Boothman and Pardee suggest that their results show a new direction for the future development of anti-cancer agents.

Throughout the history of plant medicine, practitioners – whether western herbalists or indigenous medicine men – have maintained that it is the natural extraction of the active part of the plant which has the greatest effect. Modern scientists are always seeking the 'magic bullet' of one single active principle within the complex structure of plant material. Time and time again this has been shown to be the wrong direction, as is amply demonstrated by some German research. Wagner, Kreher and Jurcic at the Institute of Pharmaceutical Biology, University of Munich, conducted a detailed and systematic study of the cytotoxic (cell-killing) ability of different compounds.

They compared pure naphthaquinones with naphthaquinone-containing extracts of plants, including lapachol. The high dose of the isolated compounds suppressed the immune system but had a lethal effect on body cells, whereas the very low concentrations of naphthaquinone in the lapachol extract had the reverse effect of stimulating the body's own natural immune defence mechanism. It is fascinating to note that this same reverse effect has been found in studies of vincristine, the anti-leukaemia drug made from the Madagascan rosy periwinkle.

The rainforest Indians have always valued Lapacho as a powerful medicine in the treatment of parasites. Lopes, Cruz, Docampo et al, working at the Department of Microbiology at the University of Rio de Janeiro, published a paper as far back as 1978 in the *Annals of Tropical Medicine and Parasitology*. They investigated the effects of lapachol on *Trypanosoma cruzi*, the parasitic protozoa that causes Chagas' disease, which in its acute form mainly affects children. In this study lapachol was shown to affect the growth, the survival and the infectiousness of *T. cruzi* adversely.

In various parts of the world holistic physicians are beginning to use Lapacho as an aid to their patients' recovery from a range of illnesses which stem from immune deficiencies. In Chronic Fatigue Syndrome, Epstein-Barr virus (a likely cause of ME) and Tired All the Time syndrome, Lapacho can be a great aid to recovery owing to its positive effects on the immune system.

There has been considerable interest in lapachol in the USA and it has been included in the anti-cancer screening programme of the National Cancer Institute. The Institute reported slight anti-tumour effects from two varieties of Lapacho, but to the best of my knowledge no further research has yet been done by the NCI. One of America's leading holistic physicians, Dr Robert Atkins, makes several references to Lapacho in his book *Dr Atkins' Health Revolution*. He describes how he uses the plant himself along with a variety of other natural medicines in the treatment of patients with severe *Candida* infections. He also refers to Dr John Parkes Trowbridge, another holistic physician working in Texas, who uses Lapacho in conjunction with homoeopathic medicines in the treatment of this yeast infection.

As yet there is no scientific evidence that Lapacho's influence on the immune system is of any help in the treatment of HIV and AIDS, but many practitioners who are attempting to treat these dreadful conditions by boosting the body's own natural defences are including Lapacho in their regimes. Australian doctor Ian Brighthope is just one holistic physician who includes Lapacho as part of his regime of various health-boosting supplements.

One of the most eminent American experts in the field of herbal medicine is Dr Paul Lee. Before becoming director of the Platonic Academy in Santa Cruz, California, he taught both at MIT and Harvard. As far back as 1988 he wrote about his own personal pro-gramme for improving natural immunity using herbs and specifi-cally included Lapacho as a valuable plant which could reduce the risks of cancer. Although there is a great deal of anecdotal evidence of the value of this rainforest plant, Lee points out that there are so far few clinical studies to which we may refer. He describes Lapacho as an immune enhancer which, although it does not improve specific immunity, increases the level of the general immune defence mechanism. 'This should be subject to scientific analysis', says Dr Lee.

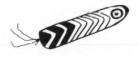

Of all the people I have met during my travels in the Amazon, one of the most exciting, enthusiastic and informative was Walter Radames Accorsi, Emeritus Professor of Botany at the University of São Paulo and founder of the Brazilian Ethnobotanical Society. This elderly academic simply oozed enthusiasm for the whole sub-ject of plant medicine and is one of the world's great experts in the application of modern scientific methods in research into tradi-tional native medicines.

Here is the real scientist who seeks the truth but whose vision is unfettered by the blinkers that restrict many academics. Accorsi is currently researching the traditional native belief in Lapacho as a treatment for various types of cancer. In collaboration with local hospitals and GPs in São Paulo he runs a free clinic where any patient with a diagnosis of cancer can come for complementary therapy using Lapacho. Although the professor repeatedly told me that his studies were still in their infancy and that no absolute conclusions could be drawn from them, several hundred case studies were beginning to show extraordinary results. In the treatment of various cancers, leukaemia and a variety of other conditions, he describes Lapacho as being of excellent therapeutic value.

Traditionally, Lapacho is used in the form of a tea or compress made from the bark, capsules and tablets for internal use, and Lapacho powder which is sprinkled on to wounds. The various chemicals in Lapacho – including alkaloids, glucosides, quinones, xyladine, tannins and especially the phenolic derivative lapachol – give this plant a variety of therapeutic values. Lapacho is analgesic, sedative, decongestant, cardiotonic, anti-haemorrhagic, diuretic, appetite stimulating, astringent, hypotensive and anti-bacterial. Consequently it is used in the treatment of cancers, leukaemia, ulcers, rheumatism, high blood-pressure, cystitis, pelvic inflammatory disease and skin diseases.

Professor Accorsi is positive that his work with cancer patients will produce the clinical test results that the folklore of the rainforest Indians predicts. But he is adamant that no claims for 'miracle cures' or 'dramatic breakthroughs' should be made in his name in the search for a cure for cancer. 'It would be unscientific, unprofessional and unfair to raise unfounded hopes in those poor people afflicted with cancer before we are certain of our results and before they have been repeated by other research workers.' These were the professor's final words to me after our fascinating day together in São Paulo.

Of all the herbs used in traditional medicine by the ancient Incas, Lapacho was one of the mainstays. In the four centuries since the Spanish conquest of the Incas, Lapacho has cropped up from time to time in Europe – Czar Nicholas II of Russia and Ghandi are known to have taken a daily morning cup of Lapacho tea.

The bark of the Lapacho tree is to this day collected from the wild and impenetrable interiors of the Brazilian forest. Now Brazilian doctors as well as the rainforest tribes use the shredded bark to make a healing brew. As research has progressed, most experts now consider that the best results are obtained by grinding the bark into a fine powder and taking it in capsules. Two to three grams a day are all that is needed to experience the healing properties of Lapacho – possibly the greatest legacy of the Incas.

Pfaffia or Brazilian Ginseng

For hundreds of years the rainforest Indians in Brazil have used the root of this plant as a cure-all. In fact the urban population of Brazil named it *para todo* – the Portuguese words meaning 'for everything'. First described by the great South American botanist Carl von Martius in the mid-1800s and later named *Pfaffia paniculata* by Kuntze, this native plant of the *Amaranthaceae* family is now botanically described as *Pfaffia paniculata (Martius) Kuntze*.

The Xingu tribe of rainforest Indians living in the Matto Grosso region of Brazil have used Pfaffia since time immemorial. But after its original description by von Martius and its definitive classification by Kuntze in 1891, it seems to have disappeared from western literature until 1975. In that year a famous Brazilian herbalist, Jair, came across a Xingu shaman or medicine man. He explained the value of Pfaffia to Jair, who was enthralled by the possibilities of this new herbal treatment. The medicine man described its use as an aphrodisiac, in the healing of wounds, in the treatment of diabetes and even for the relief of cancer. Since Pfaffia appears to be a panacea or cure-all, it has become popularly known as Brazilian Ginseng – the Latin name for Ginseng is *Panax*, which is derived from the Greek-based word 'panacea'.

Scientifically it is far from fashionable to consider any medicament as a cure-all. Sceptical doctors raise their eyebrows in horror when herbalists and other holistic practitioners talk about 'adaptogens' which come to the aid of the body's defence mechanism and seem to have a miraculous ability to cure a host of different illnesses. It is surprising how selective doctors' attitudes to drugs can be – a herb that could be effective in a dozen different conditions is nonsense, but cortisone and penicillin are fine. These products of the pharmaceutical industry are prescribed daily to millions of patients throughout the world for dozens of different ailments.

At the time that Jair found out about Pfaffia, there was a large Japanese population in Brazil. Knowing of their passionate interest in the true Ginseng – an interest encouraged by its proven ability to help combat excessive stress and its use as an aphrodisiac – he made Pfaffia available to them. The association with Ginseng was enhanced by the fact that it is the enormous root of the Pfaffia which is used in the preparation of this herbal medicine. Just like Ginseng, the root must be at least seven years old before it is used. The Japanese community in Brazil soon aroused the interest of their countrymen at home in this 'new' plant from the rainforest and it was not long before a group of Japanese researchers published a paper describing three new chemical substances which they had isolated from Pfaffia. These substances, nortriterpene saponins or pfaffocides D, E and F, all have the ability to prevent the growth of cultured tumour cells. I wonder if the Xingu tribesmen knew that?

As news of the Japanese discoveries filtered back to Brazil, it caught the attention of one of the country's leading scientists. Dr Milton Brazzach, head of the Pharmacology Department at the University of São Paulo, obtained some of the Japanese workers' original papers describing the anti-tumour activity of the pfaffocides which they had isolated. From that time on Dr Brazzach was committed to further study of this ancient rainforest medicine.

He has collected a massive quantity of detailed case histories – around three thousand in all – in which this remarkable root has been used for the treatment of cancer, diabetes, chronic fatigue syndrome, joint disorders, cholesterol reduction and even in the control of uric acid in relation to gout and arthritis.

Like its namesake, the true Ginseng, Brazilian Ginseng contains significant amounts of germanium, involved in the mechanism which delivers oxygen to the body cells. This probably accounts for the tonic and stimulating effect, but Pfaffia also contains beta-carotene, vitamins B1 and B2, vitamin E, potassium and small amounts of other minerals, and a full spectrum of the essential amino acids including arginine – recently used in trials at Great Ormond Street Hospital as a natural treatment to reverse arterial damage in arteriosclerosis.

Another surprising discovery in the make-up of Pfaffia is that of three vegetable hormones: beta-ecdysone, sitosterol and stigmasterol. Beta-ecdysone, worth around US$4,000 per gram, is a stimulant to cell growth triggering the development of new and vigorous cells. Sitosterol appears to have a beneficial effect on the reduction of blood cholesterol levels, whilst stigmasterol is a natural precursor of oestrogen. For this reason the value of Pfaffia in the treatment of menopausal symptoms is now arousing considerable interest. As an aid in reducing mood swings and hot flushes and possibly even helping to reduce the likelihood of osteoporosis, Pfaffia could provide a natural safe alternative to hormone replacement therapy, which is sometimes contra-indicated. Between 1 g and 4 g a day taken in capsule form is the usual dose.

Anyone interested in the growing and rapidly developing world of the scientific application of plant medicines will be keeping a very close eye on Pfaffia research. Will it be an active treatment for tumours? Can it produce sufficient improvement in the body's natural immune defences to protect against degenerative diseases? Is it possible that this ancient plant could even become a standard treatment for diabetes?

Only proper research and time will tell.

Catuaba

In the Brazilian state of Minas there is a proverb which says, 'Until a father reaches 60, the son is his; after that the son is Catuaba's.' Traditionally this is the most famous of all the Brazilian aphrodisiac plants, used by the indigenous population for generations.

There are two species of Catuaba, one of which is found in the northern regions of Brazil: in the Amazon, Para, Pernambuco, Bahia, Maranhão and Alagoas. Here the Catuaba tree reaches immense height and thickness, producing small yellow flowers and a dark yellow fruit. The second species is found in the central areas, growing in Espirito Santo, São Paulo and Minas Gerais. Here it forms a large bushy shrub. The species are equally effective medicinally and a traditional herbal tea is prepared from the bark. As it has a very bitter flavour the Brazilians sweeten the tea with a little honey or a product derived from another of their amazing rainforest plants, an extract of Stevia (see below). Never ones to do things by halves, the exhuberant Brazilians often mix the tea with their own lethal cane sugar brandy, cachaça.

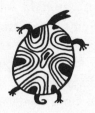

Botanically the rampant vigorous tree is known as *Erythroxylon catuaba martius*, a member of the *Eritroxilaceae* family. The Catuaba is so vigorous and strongly growing that it tends to force out other plant species and form huge forests of its own.

In his book, *Cures with Yoga and Medicinal Plants*, published in Rio in 1979, Chiang Sing says of Catuaba:

> It has been appreciated by the local populations for generations. The Tupi Indians first discovered the qualities of the plant and composed many songs praising it. The bark of the Catuaba functions as a stimulant of the nervous system, above all when one deals with functional impotence of the male genital organs. It is an innocent aphrodisiac, used without any ill side effects at all. Catuaba is a natural aphrodisiac and sexual stimulant. It is reported that after drinking three or four cups of tea steadily over a period of time, the first symptoms are usually erotic dreams and then increased sexual desire.

> Uses: influential in the treatment of sexual impotence; aphrodisiac, tonic for the genitals. (Chiang Sing, *Cura Com Yoga e Plantas Medicinais*, Freitas Bastos, Rio de Janeiro, 1979)

In spite of, or maybe because of, the wide use and enormous popularity of Catuaba, there has been little research into its chemical construction or active ingredients. The World Health Organization did institute a survey of over 120 Brazilian plants with reputed aphrodisiac properties, and Catuaba was one of only three designated for further investigation. As far as I have been able to ascertain, there are not yet any published results of this work.

Catuaba is available as capsules, but if the idea of tea is more appealing they can be opened and the powder inside can be added to boiling water, sweetened with a little honey and even spiced up a little with some alcohol. One gram morning and evening is the usual dosage. Whilst it is beneficial to men and women it is in the area of male impotence that the most striking results have been reported. There is no evidence of side-effects, even after long-term use.

Curmonsky, Napoleon's chef, once said, 'Properly speaking there are no aphrodisiacs capable of endowing those blind to life with sight. But for those with poor eyesight in this matter, there are substances which act as magnifying lenses.' Perhaps Catuaba is the magnifying glass to solve your problem.

Stevia

The consumption of sugar throughout the western world is rising at a rate so great as to cause considerable concern in medical circles. In spite of the constant protestations of the sugar industry that sugar is a 'natural' product and has no harmful effects other than the encouragement of dental decay, many clinicians are alarmed by the vast amounts of sugar consumed, especially by children. An article in the Food and Drug Administration publication (FDA) *Consumer*, April 1992, states that in America:

> According to the US Department of Agriculture data on the amount of caloric sweeteners used in food, there has been an increase of more than 16% on a per person basis over the last two decades and more than half of the increase has occurred in the last five years.

Calorific sweeteners include sugar, high fructose corn syrup, pure honey and edible syrups.

Paul Lachance, chairman of the Department of Food Science at Rutgers University in New Jersey, states this in another way. He estimates that, based on a 2,000-calorie-a-day diet, the average American consumes about three hundred calories from sugars added to food. That comes to the equivalent of nearly fourteen teaspoons of table sugar a day. According to Joan Gussow, professor of nutrition and education at Columbia Teacher's College, Columbia University, New York, 'we have developed a relentless sweet tooth, a severe addiction to sweetness'.

Could Stevia be the answer? Is it possible that there is a completely natural sweetener with absolutely no calories, that is safe for diabetics and can be used on food, in your cakes and added to drinks and won't rot your teeth? The answer is yes.

Stevia rebaudiana, Bertoni is a small shrubby plant of the *Compositae* family which grows wild throughout Brazil. This perennial shrub loses its leaves during the Brazilian winter. With the first sign of spring, there is an explosion of growth from the woody base of the shrub, which is soon a mass of leaves and flowers.

The Indians living close to Brazil's southern border with Paraguay have used Stevia for thousands of years. Their name for this extraordinary shrub is kaa-hee. They used the leaves of the plant to add sweetness to their food and drinks. The great explorer and botanist Bertoni was the first western scientist to discover the properties of Stevia and brought its attention to the western world. The *Kew Bulletin* published in 1901 gave us the first description of this plant and the Indians' use of it.

Stevia is three hundred times sweeter than sugar and the chemical substance which produces this sweetness is stevioside. This is a glycoside molecule comprising glycose and an aglycide known as esteviol. Stevioside is not found in the roots of the plant, there is little in the wood and small quantities are found in the flowers. It is the leaves of the plant which are the real source of this extraordinary sweetness, stevioside accounting for around 10% of the dry weight of the leaves. The traditional way in which Stevia is used is by infusing the dried leaf together with other herbal or Indian teas – just a leaf or two in the pot produces a brew to satisfy the sweetest tooth. Alternatively the leaves can be steeped in boiling water for ten minutes and strained; the liquid is then used as a sweetener. Modern technology allows us to extract the stevioside and dry it into a fine white powder or granules which can be used from a bowl just like sugar.

There have been many scientific studies of Stevia – at the University of Bangkok; Lehman College of Biological Sciences, New York; the Department of Physiology and Medical Sciences, University of São Paulo, Brazil; the Department of Pharmacology, University of São Paulo, Brazil; the Department of Odontology, University of São Paulo; and other research establishments in Holland, America and Japan. All these studies show Stevia to be safe and without side-effects. One of the experiments even demonstrated a protective effect against tooth decay due to the tannin content of the leaves. Stevia has been found to increase glucose tolerance in normal adult human beings and it significantly reduced the levels of blood glucose during the test and after overnight fasting. This research would appear to support the traditional Brazilian view that Stevia could be helpful in the treatment of diabetes.

As recently as the summer of 1992, *Herbalgram*, the education publication of the American Botanical Council, carried a report about the US FDA ordering companies to stop using Stevia and prohibiting its importation. In his article, Mark Blumentahl reports that the American Herbal Products Association had written to FDA commissioner Dr David Kessler, asking him to agree that Stevia should be recognised as GRAS (Generally Recognised As Safe) as a food and that it is not, as the FDA had contended, a food additive. The AHPA submitted two hundred pages of documentation detailing the history of safe food use as well as further scientific safety data on Stevia from a formal safety review carried out by Professor Douglas A. Kinghorn for the Herb Research Foundation. The AHPA filed a formal GRAS petition on 24 April 1992.

Stevia is widely used throughout the world and has been used continuously for hundreds of years in Brazil. Japanese food manufacturers use it, as do other Asian and European producers. I am never sure that it is good practice to encourage the sweet tooth habit, but for those who must have sweetness, Stevia is a natural, no-calorie, no-side-effect, no-after-taste and no-risk substitute for tooth-rotting, fattening and consequently heart-disease-encouraging sugar.

Epilogue

A final plea for conservation and biodiversity

At the time I came back from my first trip to the Amazonian rain-forest at the end of 1988, I was writing a weekly column for one of the national women's magazines. Naturally I wrote a full description of my eye-opening visit to Brazil. At the front of the magazine the editor's weekly letter appears. To coincide with the issue that contained my article this is what she said:

Advice from the Amazon

I'm sure practically half the northern hemisphere were aware of complementary health correspondent Michael van Straten's trip up the Amazon. Every time he phoned or came to see us he managed to drop it casually into the conversation. Then, when he returned, we were treated to minute by minute accounts of the food, the scenery and the people he met. It was fascinating, of course – the only reason I mention him going on about it is that we were all unashamedly jealous. Michael was there to work, however. On page 42 you can read his article about the lifestyle of the people living in the innermost reaches of this gargantuan river. It seems that despite – or maybe because of – their poverty, they can still teach us a thing or two about natural ways to preserve our health.

Since then there has been a continuous stream of publicity about the rainforest and the way in which human greed is despoiling it. There have been major conferences on environment, ecology and biodiversity, yet still the gold diggers pour their mercury into the Amazon, the wood industry fells the trees and the cattle barons burn hundreds of thousands of acres of virgin forest. All this is in the name of 'progress', but in reality it is a matter of greed. Around the world, rainforest which would cover the size of Scotland disappears each year.

Putting on one side the potential revenue from plant-derived medicines, the revenue per hectare from rubber and Brazil nuts is four times the revenue from cattle ranching. We cannot afford to disregard this huge but rapidly vanishing treasure trove of plants potentially useful to mankind, both as foods and medicines. Neither can we ignore the needs of biodiversity, since to preserve the plants we must preserve the habitat and within the rainforest there is great interdependence of species. The Brazil nut, for instance, requires the orchid bee to fertilise it – no orchids, no orchid bee; no orchid bee, no Brazil nut. When the nut finally falls to the ground the only animal that can penetrate its hard shell and release the nut is the agouti, a rainforest rodent. Without the agouti there would be no dispersion of the Brazil nut tree.

We must never give up the fight to protect the world we live in, but there is also another fight – the fight to overcome prejudice and blinkered attitudes towards herbal medicines. In the spring of 1993 there appeared to be an organised attack in the American media claiming that herbal medicines were unregulated and unsafe and that claims for their effectiveness were unsubstantiated. This is just not true. There are libraries full of scientific studies describing the benefits and safety of herbal medicines. There are strict government controls in Europe, the UK and the USA over all medicines and claims made for them. One does not wish to look for consipiracies. The fact is that public disquiet with many of the products of the giant pharmaceutical companies is leading people to vote with their feet and turn to the often gentler and safer remedies from nature.

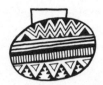

It would be a fool who denied the massive benefits of the modern pharmaceutical industry to mankind. Consider life without anaesthetics, antibiotics, hormones, anti-cancer drugs and painkillers. But is the pharmaceutical industry getting nervous? Is it worried about natural remedies which cannot be patented and cannot earn them billions of dollars?

Just to put the safety question into perspective, in 1989 in the USA there were 140 accidental deaths through anti-depressants, 126 through analgesics, 78 through sedatives and 70 through heart drugs. These were not deliberate overdoses but deaths caused by proper use of these four major categories of drugs, all of which are licensed, approved and considered safe. In the same year there was one death reported as a result of plant poisoning.

The Herb Research Foundation in Boulder, Colorado, has searched the National Library of Medicines database covering international medical and scientific literature over the last thirty years. They have also studied the reports of the American Association of Poison Control Centers and they found no substantial evidence that herbs are causing toxicity problems. Herbs have been used by humans for thousands of years, and the World Health Organization is actively encouraging the use of traditional forms of medicine in developing countries. WHO issued guidelines stating:

> A guiding principle should be, if the product has been traditionally used without demonstrated harm, no specific restrictive regulatory action should be undertaken unless

new evidence demands a revised risk – benefit assessment …
Prolonged and apparently uneventful use of a substance usually offers testimony of its safety.

Finally, we need to worry about our own backyard as well as the
world's dwindling rainforests. It is probable that European and
North American forests are vanishing faster than those in Brazil.
During the past fifty years 45% of our finest woods have vanished
or been decimated, compared with 10% of the Amazonian forest
that has been felled.

It is my fervent hope that this small book will convey a sense of
my excitement and enthusiasm at discovering some of the wonders
of the rainforest. Science has merely scratched the tip of this extraordinary iceberg and 90% of the flora in the Amazon has never
been studied to determine its chemical composition. The
Amazonian Indians are often the only ones who understand the
properties of their own forest plants and how they are best used.
This knowledge must be an essential part of every effort to conserve
and preserve the rainforest.

Index